THE WALLS OF SALVATION: THE DUALITAS

THE WALLS OF SALVATION: THE DUALITAS

IN ALL THINGS…..FRANK'S STORY

AN ADULT CHRISTIAN NOVEL

BY

JOHN MICHAEL TOSTI

INVITATION: PLEASE VISIT OUR WEBSITES FOR INFORMATION ABOUT THE AUTHOR'S FIRST NOVEL, *THE BOOK OF ITTAI*

TheBookofIttai.com and SwordofGoliath.com

ISBN 978-0-557-84906-2

TABLE OF CONTENTS

PREFACE

Matthew 8:1-3 tells us: When he came down from the mountainside, large crowds followed him. A man with leprosy came and knelt before him and said, "Lord, if you are willing, you can make me clean." Jesus reached out his hand and touched the man. "I am willing," he said. "Be clean!" Immediately he was cured of his leprosy.

In 2 Corinthians 12:7-9 Paul tells us about praying to be healed of his own physical ailment: To keep me from becoming conceited because of these surpassingly great revelations, there was given me a thorn in my flesh, a messenger of Satan, to torment me. Three times I pleaded with the Lord to take it away from me. But he said to me, "My grace is sufficient for you, for my power is made perfect in weakness."

How does a Christian who is suffering from a serious physical or mental illness come to terms with the Jesus who says, "I am willing," "Be clean!" And the same Jesus who says, "My grace is sufficient for you, for my power is made perfect in weakness."

I think the answer is found in Romans 8:28: "And we know that in all things God works for the good of those who love him, who have been called according to his purpose."

This book, *The Walls of Salvation: The Dualitas*, is the story of a man named Frank "Sonny" Angelo. Frank suffered half of his life with a progressive form of Multiple Sclerosis. His story is a testament to God's transforming power and an embodiment of Romans 8:28: "And we know that in all things God works for the good of those who love him, who have been called according to his purpose."

This book is based on a true story. We meet Frank at the lowest point in his life. Multiple Sclerosis has destroyed his body. Living in a poorly funded public nursing home, he has no movement left in his body save the ability to slightly turn his head. He has been devoted to Jesus for most of the last twenty years and has lived by the Lord's promise that, "My grace is sufficient for you for my power is made perfect in weakness." In a moment of despair, Frank gives in to self pity and questions God. He cries out, "Why God? Why did you make me live like this?" He wonders what his life might have been like, if only he had not gotten sick. "If only," those words of lament so commonly used by one in despair.

God hears Frank's plea and grants him a glimpse of the life he might have had, if only... We then see the duality of man, the flesh versus the spirit.

A man spends most of his adult life as an invalid. He doesn't hold a job, lives without a wife, has minimal contact with his children and regarded by the world as someone to pity. He is the kind of person those of us who have our health and strength see and think, "I'm glad that's not me." But in reality, how does God view this man who suffers for twenty years but continues praising Him and telling people about Jesus. Is his life a tragedy or a triumph?

God has a great plan for His children. The plan and design is so grand and so intricate that we cannot possibly understand it. We see pieces of the plan and we know how our lives affect others to a degree but can we truly understand the impact our lives have on others? I don't think we can, but God understands, and he has interwoven the fabric of our lives with so many others according to His great design. "The Walls of Salvation: The Dualitas," explores how one man can impact many others for bad if he rejects God or ultimately for good if he is willing to trust and obey God no matter the circumstances in his life.

THE WALLS OF SALVATION

The Walls of Salvation, which side are you on?

The Walls of Salvation, protection or denial,

The Walls of Salvation, which side are you on?

The Walls of Salvation, acceptance or disavowal,

The Walls of Salvation, which side are you on?

The Walls of Salvation, on this question you must dwell.

The Walls of Salvation, which side are you on?

The Walls of Salvation, the answer determines Heaven or Hell.

ABOUT THE AUTHOR – John M. Tosti

In my first book, "The Book of Ittai", I did not include any notes about myself for several reasons. First, I felt that anything about me would take away from the authentic feel of the imagined found manuscript. Second, if forced to describe myself in this context I would only say, "His accomplishments have been few and his sins have been many." However, some people, who I respect, told me that they thought a note about the author would have enhanced my first book. So in deference to their wisdom I will include the following.

I was born in Albany, New York, the setting for this book, in 1949. I graduated from St. Bernard College in 1971. My wife and I have been married for thirty years and have four sons and three grandchildren with a fourth on the way. I have been involved as a local businessman in Birmingham, Alabama for the past thirty years. Although raised a Catholic, I didn't come to know the Lord until I was age forty-two. The Lord started to deal with me at age forty and I fought hard before surrendering two years later. During a particularly difficult phase of my life, I was sitting in my bedroom depressed and commiserating to myself about just how bad life was. Out of the blue, a Bible Verse flashed into my mind. It was Deuteronomy 2:7. Please know that at this time I was not well read in the Bible and didn't even know where Deuteronomy was located in the book. It was so clear and persistent that I immediately found an unused Bible we had somewhere in the house and read the following;

> "The Lord your God has blessed you in all the work of
> your hands. He has watched over your journey through
> this vast desert. These forty years the Lord your God
> has been with you, and you have not lacked anything."
> Deuteronomy 2:7

Well, that was a wake-up call and I had to concede that compared to how most of the residents on this planet live, I indeed had it pretty good despite my so-called difficult circumstances at the time.

Over the years I have tried to serve the Lord in various ministries and have had some minor successes and many miserable failures in my walk with the Lord. I am eternally grateful for the following word from God:

> "Then Peter came to Jesus and asked, 'Lord, how many times shall I forgive my brother when he sins against me? Up to seven times?" Jesus answered, "I tell you, not seven times, but seventy-seven times."(Mt. 18:21–22)

At the risk of seeming to come across as too mystical, I have been blessed with strong leadings or influences from the Holy Spirit over the years. Much of this book, as well as the previous book came about with His help. I've been amazed how often I would receive ideas or phrases from "out of the blue," to complete a thought, a page or chapter when I have gotten stuck while in the process of writing. St Francis of Assisi said, "I have been all things unholy. If God can work through me, He can work through anyone." It is with tremendous gratitude to God that I acknowledge how applicable that quotation is to my life.

Fearing that I am becoming self-indulgent, I'll say no more about the author other than to say that my goal in writing this book is to bring glory to God, bless the reader and honor the memory of my father.

DEDICATION

This book is dedicated to the memory of my father Frank Tosti whose life was dedicated to the Lord Jesus Christ.

SPECIAL THANKS

Special thanks to my Uncle and brother in Christ, Tom Patterson, for his insights into my father's life and for the many kindnesses that he and his wife Marcia showed me in my youth.

Special thanks to my mother, Rita Hulett, for sharing some memories and anecdotes of my father. You always did your best and I am forever grateful.

Special thanks to my wife, Hazel, for being my inspiration and for helping me navigate this thing we call life. I would be lost without you.

PROLOGUE

What's wrong with me? I am so tired and yet I can't get to sleep. The strength I once had is all but gone. I'm ill tempered and can't think of anything else but the numbness in my hands and feet. This waiting for them to tell me just how sick I am and that I'm going to die is intolerable. Maybe I should drive down to the Dunn Memorial Bridge and jump into the Hudson River and kill myself. Maybe that is the answer.

Wallowing in my self-pity, I finally found some relief in sleep. My reality becomes a dense forest and I find myself walking down a hard dirt path. It's nighttime, it's cold and I am alone. My way is lit only by the moon and stars. I happen onto a small cottage. The flickering of a warm fire and candlelight becomes visible through a small front window and invites me to walk up to the door and knock to seek its promise of shelter and security. I knock and this old man, a priest, gray and stooped by his many years, answers the door.

"Welcome my son. Come in out of the cold. I've been expecting you." He said, urging me to enter with a gesture of his gnarled hand.

I followed him into the entrance of the cottage that leads to his study. Stacks of aged, leather-bound books filled a credenza behind his small davenport desk. I remained silent and strangely felt no need to speak as I sensed this is what the priest expected of me. The old man's kindly manner and the soft light of his fire and the candles created an atmosphere of peace and acceptance. Walking to the credenza, he examined several of the books before choosing one. Then he sat down into a comfortable chair and pulled himself up to his desk. Opening the book, he licked his thumb and began leafing through the pages; he looked up and invited me to have a seat on a wooden chair located in front of his desk.

He began to speak, "Frank my son, yes, I know your name. I know everything about you. It's all right here in this book. This book is the story of your life and it contains two narratives. As you can see there is no front or back cover, they are both the same. Look closely; there is script on both sides of each leaf within the book. If you open the book from this end, it tells your story as it will be. If you open the book from the opposite end, it tells your story as it may be. In his infinite wisdom, God will decide your life's path and the outcome of your book.

On the edge of his desk, there was an hourglass with most of the grains of sand still filling the top portion of the device. Slowly but inevitably grain by grain fell to the bottom of the glass. Then suddenly the grains began to rush through from the top to the bottom of the timepiece. It was as if an avalanche of time was flooding through the narrow passage joining the top and bottom of the timepiece. The sight of this alarmed me so much that the priest raised his hand in a calming gesture and said, "Be still and I will explain the meaning of the hourglass."

The priest moved the hourglass in front of him. His touch seemed to slow the movement of the sand. He began to speak. "Frank, what you see before you represents how you live your life. Man's life on earth is but a handbreadth according to eternity. Time is a precious commodity. Spend it wisely and the grains of sand move slowly but waste it and the sands of your life flow quickly as a river in flood stage. If you waste your life seeking your own personal gratification, how will anything of lasting value truly be accomplished?"

The priest stood and walked around his desk and stood over me. Placing his hand on my shoulder he said, "My son, you must go now. You are about to begin a journey that you do not wish to undertake. However, be faithful and strong, live for the Lord, and bring him glory, and your reward will be great."

PART I

WHAT WAS

CHAPTER 1

MISERY

I've been lying in my filth for at least two hours. Why doesn't the nurse come and check on me? When she finally comes, she'll curse at me for soiling this bed and making her have to clean my mess. Dear Lord, if I must have MS, must I also endure all this shame? For over twenty years I've been on my back unable to move. I can hardly turn my neck and don't even have the strength to speak above a whisper. If I call out for help no one hears me. The mucous is building up in my windpipe and needs to be suctioned. Breathing at all is most difficult. If my nose itches I can't scratch it and if I have a bowel movement before they bring the bedpan, then I just lay here in my own filth choking on this foul odor. Rarely does anyone come to visit me. I have nothing but you Lord and you are enough…. But Lord, I don't understand why I have had to live this life.

It was bearable when I was able to live at home. My mother, God bless her, took such good care of me. For these twenty years she was there for me day and night. She loves me so much, but since her strength and money ran out, it became impossible for her, so they moved me to this county home for invalids. Now I'm lucky if they check on me more than a few times a day. When my mother was able to care for me I almost never had a bedsore and now they tell me my backside is covered with them. All I have is you Lord and you have always been enough to get me through, but even so, these last few months in this home have been too much. Lord, you said that you would not put more on us than we are able to bear. Well, I've reached my breaking point. This is all too much for me to carry. Please take my life now, I cannot endure another day. Your word says that you are a merciful God. If your word is true then please have mercy on me.

How many times have I prayed to you to heal me? You healed the invalid at the pool of Bethesda but you have not healed me! Why Lord, why! The elders have anointed me with oil many times and begged you to heal me but you have not responded. We have the faith! I believe in you! My youth has been stolen from me. My wife and children have long ago abandoned me. So here I am lying in my own filth unable to move a muscle. I have no resources. I have nothing but I still cling to my faith in you. Answer me! I am begging you for mercy! Show me why I have had to live this way. Show me why I have had to suffer this much. You are God. All is under your control. The Bible talks about restoration. Restore my life! Give me back my life! Could I have not served you better with strong limbs? Reached more people with your word if I could shout your message? Hear me, please, please....!

Suddenly, Nurse Perkins burst into my room, "Frank! Frank! What have you done? Have you messed your bed again? I know you have, I can smell it! Now I have to clean it and me with my bad back. You ain't worth spit, do you know that! You're just good for nothin'. I'm about to go off my shift, I'll just leave you for the night nurse. Maybe you'll learn. I know you can hold it if you wanted to." Nurse Perkins stormed off leaving me to wallow in my filth and hoping, I guess, someone else would clean me.

Is that the answer to my prayers? I began to sob and started to choke on my own my tears. I passed out. At least when I am unconscious I'm not aware of my circumstances. In my unconscious state my life and the years of my trials flashed into my mind. I found myself back working with my partner Tommy Phelan. Tommy and I were in the scrap metal business. It was only a few years after the war and there was a demand for scrap and dealers were paying a premium for anything we brought in. Tommy and I were boyhood friends, growing up in Albany's south end. His family was the only Irish family on Herkimer Street. He was a great partner. Not only did we always see eye to eye about the business, but at 6 feet tall, he weighed at least 300 lbs and could lift a ton of scrap. Tommy saw action in the Pacific during the war. I was so proud of him. Unfortunately, due to my club foot, all the branches of the service refused to take me, even the Coast Guard. I did what I could here at home, but not serving during the war was one of the biggest disappointments of my life. It was helping out with the various war drives that led me to the scrap business. When Tommy got home, I knew he would be the perfect partner.

We went in together 50/50 and bought a 1945 Ford flatbed truck. A friend of ours who was a carpenter, Carlo Crishone, built us wooden slats to attach to the flatbed. This let us carry some heavy hauls of scrap and saved us a lot of time. By 1953 we were making pretty good money. Tommy and I both pulled down $250 to $300 every week. In fact, business had been so good that me and my wife Rosie were looking to buy our own house.

I married Rosie in 1948. The next year we had a son, Ricardo. The following year, my two boys from my first marriage, Bobby and Frank Jr, came to live with us. Their mother said that they would either go live with me or they had to go to the LaSalle home for boys. She just couldn't or wouldn't be a mother. So there I was, 26 years old with a wife and three boys, making good money, looking to buy a house. I was doing pretty darn well. In fact, so well, Tommy and I decided that we would only have to work the scrap business another year or so and then we would have enough saved to buy a bar. This was our dream. It would be more of a night club. We would serve booze of course, specialize in Italian food and have live entertainment. The south end of Albany, where we lived, was loaded with talent. That's where most of the Italians, Jews and coloreds lived and let me tell you, there were many very good musicians, singers and dancers looking for a break. It didn't matter to us if you where black or white, we all got along, maybe because of the hard times that most of us went through. Life for working class people in the south end of Albany was day to day.

As for me, I loved to sing. In 1947 I won second place in the Frank Sinatra contest at the Palace Theatre over on Pearl Street. I should have won that contest too. Everyone told me I had the best voice. However, the guy who won dressed just like Sinatra and basically did an impression of ole blue eyes. I remember a time when we were over Rosie's grandmother's house on Easter Sunday. Her grandmother knew I could sing and she asked me to sing the Lord's Prayer. After I finished singing, there wasn't a dry eye in the place. If I was a club owner, I'd have a place to sing every week and who knows what that might lead to. Maybe I'd have a shot at getting on Godfrey's Talent Scouts.

We lived in the top floor apartment of a three floor row house on Herkimer Street. My uncles Carlo and Peter lived on the other two floors with their families. Peter was my mother's baby brother and only a few months older than I was. We grew up together and he was more of a brother than an uncle. Peter and his wife Estelle had two daughters and a son. The boy had cerebral palsy and was in very bad condition. This made life very difficult for them. The doctors recommended that Peter and Estelle put little Mikey in a home, but they would never consider doing that. I really felt sorry for them. I remember thinking that "I'm glad I wasn't like poor little Mikey." I loved living in the old neighborhood so close to family but with my wife and three boys, we really needed more room. Thanks to the scrap business it looked like we could afford a bigger house.

So there I was working with my friend Tommy. That day really stands out for me. "Sonny, what's wrong with you today? That fridge wasn't that heavy. Why are you breathing so hard? Did Ricardo keep you and Rosie up last night?" Tommy asked.

Everyone always called me Sonny in the neighborhood because of the way my mother doted on me. I replied, "I don't know what it is. The last couple of weeks or so I haven't felt as strong, I'm always tired and my toes and fingers feel numb. Maybe I'm coming down with something or maybe it's a pinched nerve? And lately I've been having this weird dream. I haven't been sleeping well at all."

"Weird dreams, what do you mean?" Tommy questioned.

"Well, it's hard to describe. In my dream it's nighttime and I'm alone in this strange forest and see this little cottage. I go up to the door and knock and this old man, a priest, answers the door. He tells me crazy things that I don't understand. Maybe I need to stop eating so much at night? Like I said, weird dreams," I explained.

"Well, if that keeps up and you don't start feeling better you should go see the doctor," advised Tommy

Things didn't improve. I grew weaker and had no energy. I became very irritable and snapped at Rosie and the kids all the time and over nothing. My feet and hands were numb and I got dizzy for no apparent reason. It was difficult working. Thank God for Tommy. He was not only pulling his own weight in the business but mine as well. He never complained. Rosie made an appointment for me to see Dr. Paduka. His office was in the neighborhood. He had been the local family doctor for years and just about everybody depended on him.

"What do you think is wrong with me Doc?" I asked him, hoping he would tell me that all was well, that I just had a virus or a pinched nerve and would be fine in a week or so. In my heart I knew I was really sick and that something was bad wrong.

"Sonny, I don't know for sure. I have my suspicions but I don't want to be premature with a diagnosis. I want you to see a friend of mine, Dr. Macumber. He's a specialist at Albany Medical Center. I'll call him and set up a time for you to meet with him. They can run the proper tests at the hospital and maybe we can figure this out and come up with a treatment." Dr Paduka explained, doing his best to reassure me and calm my fears.

My mother, father and Rosie were all upset and worried. It didn't help that I had to wait for a couple of weeks until Albany Medical Center and Dr. Macumber could see me. I wasn't improving at all, if anything, with all the worries and stress, I seemed to grow weaker every day. Finally, the day came to meet with Dr. Macumber. He seemed very interested in helping me and put me through a battery of tests. He sent me home and told me to rest and come back next week when he would have the results of the tests. He refused to guess as to what my problem was.

Waiting for word from Dr Macumber was hell. Finally, ten days later we received a call from his office asking us to come in to discuss my condition. Rosie and I were led to the doctor's back office. He stood as we entered and asked us to take a seat as he sat down on his plush leather chair behind his large mahogany desk. Leaning forward and looking very somber he began, "Sonny, Rosie, I'm afraid I have some bad news....."

Bad news indeed, Dr. Macumber went on to explain his diagnosis, the worst case scenario, that both he and Dr. Paduka feared, Multiple Sclerosis, MS. How I came to hate that name. My body's immune system was eating away at the protective sheath that covered my nerves. This interfered with the communication between my brain and the rest of my body. Over time, this would result is deterioration of my nerves and the damage was not reversible. He said that MS had several forms and it appeared that I had the worst kind. The doctor said the disease was progressive and the immediate symptoms would include many of the things I was already experiencing, numbness, dizziness, tremors, irritability, and weakness, partial or even complete loss of sight. Eventually, he explained, I would be in a wheel chair and maybe even bedridden. There was no known cure.

At age 26, I was handed a death sentence that would be long, drawn out and get progressively worse and take 25 years to kill me. I looked over at my wife and she was crying. Rosie was younger than me and was only 22 years old. Not only was she responsible for our three year old son and my five and seven year old boys that weren't even hers, but now she would have an invalid husband to care for. What could be going on in her mind? This wasn't exactly what she had signed on for. What would we do for money? My mother and father were tailors and made a very meager living. Rosie's father had been dead ten years and her mother worked in a factory and she couldn't help. That day, the day we got the bad news, was the worst day of my life. There was so much uncertainty, so much emotional pain that I couldn't control myself and threw up right there in Dr. Macumber's office.

The doctor told me that in the beginning at least, I might have some good days and if they came, I should make the most of them because later on there would not be a good day. He told me I needed to quit smoking and drinking, as that would only make matters worse. He gave us a name and phone number of a person who might be able to help us with public assistance. Welfare… I couldn't believe that my family would have to go on welfare. Dr. Macumber said, "Sonny, this isn't your fault. There is no shame in letting the government help you. You have to think about Rosie and the kids."

I knew he was right. What else could I do? Maybe the doctors are wrong, they're not always right. I remember my Uncle Fabio, the doctors told him he had six months to live and he's still alive and that was over five years ago. No, I will not give up, they can't be right.

CHAPTER 2

LOSING EVERYTHING

I didn't get better. Oh yeah, there were a few days here and there that I did actually feel ok, but with each passing month those good days were fewer and shorter. I tried to work for a while, but I just couldn't continue the heavy manual labor that the scrap business required. It wasn't fair to Tommy. He agreed to pay me $200 each week for two months for my share in the Ford but after that he couldn't afford to pay me anymore as he had to hire a helper. Even Tommy wasn't strong enough to lift some of those old appliances by himself.

The numbness in my hands and feet grew worse, my hands would shake uncontrollably at times, which was very embarrassing, I was dizzy a lot and one of my greatest fears, I was losing my sight. My vision would come and go, not completely, some days it was like being in constant twilight and some days I would be alright. Needless to say, I was no longer able to drive a car. That fact hit me hard. My independence was gone.

Within a few months of receiving the diagnosis, I needed a cane to walk. One year later I needed a wheelchair. I no longer had the strength in my legs to stand. I was constantly losing my temper, yelling at Rosie and the kids. She and I fought all the time. The money issue really added to all the problems. We were behind on the rent and the little we got from Welfare was not nearly enough for a family of five. The dream of owning our own house was a distant memory. We went through our savings in a year. This was going to be the down payment on our house. Friends and family would bring food to help us out. The most difficult thing was realizing that our situation would not get better. We were without hope.

One day my irritability and moodiness got the best of me. There was a couple who lived next door to us on Herkimer Street named Pete and Bonnie Cirullo. Bonnie was Rosie's best friend. My youngest, Ricardo and their son Jimmy, both four years old, were playmates.

I don't know how it happened but somehow while Ricardo and Jimmy were playing in the backyard, Jimmy got his nose broken. I heard these screams coming from outside. I looked out the window and Bonnie was running with little Jimmy in her arms. His face was a bloody mess. Rosie ran outside to help and brought Bonnie and Jimmy into our kitchen. Rosie quickly wet a towel and held it to Jimmy's nose trying to stop the bleeding. It was a terrible scene. Blood was gushing from his nose. Ricardo was standing in the corner looking terrified and embarrassed. I know he didn't mean to hurt Jimmy and he felt terrible. With all the commotion going on, my little son came over to me and said, "Well Dad, I guess I showed Jimmy." I think he just didn't know what else to say. I lost it and slapped my four year old son across his little face so hard that I left welts on his check. He started to cry and had this look on his face asking why I would do this to him. I hated that I did that.

On top of all this, my middle boy, Frank Jr., was always getting into trouble. He was only in first grade but he was terrorizing the other kids in his class. Once he stole money from his teacher's purse when she stepped out of the room. Another time, somehow he managed to bring matches from the house to school and tried to light a fire in the school cloak room. He got suspended and sent home for a week. In hindsight, Frank Jr. had been dealt a rotten hand. His own mother didn't want him, his step mother couldn't cope with him and now, all I did was scream at him. Is it any wonder he wanted some attention even if it was negative.

With money so tight and my health growing progressively worse and all the fighting, my relationship with Rosie was on the rocks. She came to me with tears in her eyes and said, "Sonny, I can't handle all this, I can't do it all and take care of Frank Jr. and Bobby. We have no money, you need more and more care. I'm sorry but Bobby and Frankie have to go, we have to send them to LaSalle, I'm so sorry."

Rosie was still just a girl, only 23 years old. Do I wish she could have been stronger…yes? Do I blame her…no? We made arrangements with LaSalle Home for Boys to take my two older sons. I comforted myself by saying that they would only be thirty minutes away and that the Jesuit Brothers would care for them, but it broke my heart.

I called my mother and father and asked them to drive the boys to LaSalle. They wanted to love the boys but always questioned whether they were even mine. My parents always hated my first wife and suspected her of cheating on me and because of this they resented the boys and never truly opened their hearts up to them. As I said, these kids were dealt a bad hand. In my heart, however, I knew that they were my sons.

The day my mother and father came to pick up the boys was a day I'll never forget. Bobby and Frankie did not want to leave. They were desperate to stay with us. We were their family and we were sending them away. In their minds we were abandoning them. They screamed and cried something terrible. I have had nightmares hearing their screams. "Please Daddy, please, don't let them take us away!" The cries and pleading was relentless. Frankie in particular fought as hard as a 6 year old could. Screaming and crying, he held on to the leg of the kitchen table. He must have thought that if he fought hard enough we would let him stay. It took twenty agonizing minutes for my parents to finally drag the boys out of the apartment. They continued to cry and scream all the way down the three flights of stairs and into my father's car. It was agonizing for all of us. Rosie was devastated and she blamed herself for either not being able to care for them or perhaps not wanting to care for two boys that were not her own blood, especially Frankie who was always getting into trouble.

After they left, I would only see the boys a few times each year. I was just too sick to make the effort required to be with them. I relied on a relative to get the boys and then drive them back to LaSalle. I loved seeing them but with my illness I wasn't able to be a real dad. Other dads could go to the park and play catch with their sons, I couldn't.

My next trial came a few months after the boys moved to LaSalle when my wife left me and took our baby boy, Ricardo. I can't say that I was surprised. We had been fighting ever since I got sick. In fairness to her, one of the symptoms of MS is mood swings and irritability and I had that in spades. Add to that the money problems and the fact that I no longer had any sexual appetite plus her guilt over the two older boys and this young woman of 23 had enough to call it quits. Even so, I was devastated. I'm not very proud of this but after Rosie and Ricardo left, I had my Uncle Peter help me down stairs to the front stoop of our building. I sat there with my cane in hand for several hours crying. By crying I mean bawling out loud. I guess I just needed the sympathy from the neighbors. I needed somebody to be concerned and care about me, talk about self pity.

Around this time, I actually started to feel better and stronger. Dr. Macumber said that I might have periods of remission. I started to believe that I was going to get better. In my arrogance, I decided that I was ready to start dating again. After all, Rosie left me and I was only human. Rosie's brother Pat would occasionally work for me in the scrap business. He was about ten years younger than me. Pat came around to see how I was doing and I actually had the nerve to ask him to fix me up with some girls that he knew. I thought that if he knew someone I could date, then great. If not, he might go back and tell Rosie and it might make her jealous. Neither of those two things happened. My remission was short lived and before long I was weaker than ever.

When Rosie left, I could no longer maintain the apartment or manage to care for myself. My mother, God bless her, insisted that I come and live with her and my father. They had a small second story apartment above the Concino's Bakery on Pearl Street. It was only a one bedroom apartment but she was able to get a donated hospital bed and put it in her living room. I hated that she had to do this, but with no money there were no other options. For the next twenty years my mother would care for me. She was devoted to me and all else in her life took a back seat to my needs. She fed me, cleaned me, changed my sheets every day, she brushed my teeth and all with a loving attitude.

Before I got sick I was a handsome strapping man, 6 feet tall and a muscular 180 lbs. My hair was thick and I had beautiful teeth. My mother would always ask me to smile for our friends and family to show off my beautiful straight teeth. I took great pride in my appearance. Now, my muscles had atrophied and I probably only weighed about 145 lbs. My once thick dark hair was buzzed off, as it made it much easier to keep clean and groomed. The only thing I still had was my teeth and my mother would still ask me to smile to show off my pretty straight teeth. I guess that was something.

CHAPTER 3

THE SEED

They say that time goes faster as you grow older. Not so when you have MS. As my condition deteriorated, so did my ability to function day to day in a normal way. Getting in and out of my wheelchair, to use the bathroom, to bathe, to dress, now required assistance. Those few times that I was able to leave the house, great preparations had to be made. Two men had to be available to carry me down the stairs of my parents' second floor apartment and then lift me from the chair to the back seat of my parents' car. I remember a time that we drove to Rosie's mother's apartment to pick up Ricardo. Bobby and Frankie were at the LaSalle Boys' Home Summer Camp. The plan was to pick up Ricardo and then drive the thirty minutes outside of Albany to the camp. It was one of the last times the three brothers would ever be together. My mother's brother-in-law, Charlie and my Uncle Peter got me into the car. We got to the camp in good time but I was unable to get out of the car. My visit with the two older boys lasted all of five minutes. They were anxious to take Ricardo, who was now 6 years old, swimming. I sat in the car by myself for two hours. My mother had to go with the boys in order to watch them. I had to use my bed pan three times and hoped no one would see me urinate. The hardest part was listening to all the kids yelling and squealing in delight as they swam and had summer fun. All I could do was listen to the fun and wish that somehow I could be part of the activities.

Life was becoming increasingly hard and I was without hope. I became very depressed. As with most people who found themselves in my hopeless situation, I turned to God for answers. And being a good Catholic boy, I asked my mother to talk to the parish priest. The Church was always talking about miracles and I really needed a miracle. The good Father Handley said he would pray for me but as an ex-communicant, I had to do penance to pay for my sins. I was married to my first wife in the Church. We got divorced but the church considered that civil action non-binding. Rosie and I were married by a Justice of the Peace. The Church didn't recognize that union and viewed our living arrangement as Father Handley put it, "living in sin." In fact, according to the Church, my little son Ricardo was a bastard. He tried to sound sympathetic but his attitude was one of, you made your bed and now you'll have to sleep in it. My mother and father never set foot inside a Catholic Church again after that.

My mother's younger sister, my Aunt Camille, had left the Catholic Church a few years earlier and started going to a new kind of church. They called it a Pentecostal church. It was the New Albany Church of God. We use to joke and call them "Holy Rollers" because of their emotional style of worship. I had seen a few television programs that would come on early Sunday morning with this fellow named Oral Roberts and another one named Billy Graham. They preached a different Gospel than the one the priests and nuns taught us. Indeed, what they preached was entirely from the Bible unlike the Catholic Church. Not that the Catholics didn't refer to the Bible, they did from time to time, it was that the Bible was secondary to the Church's teaching and their rules and regulations. Whatever the Pope said carried more weight than the Bible. My Aunt Camille told us that the New Albany Church of God really was not about religion but about a relationship with Jesus Christ. She said that one could ask Jesus to come into their heart and receive the Holy Spirit. This was all very strange to me but exciting at the same time. It's hard to explain but I was a little frightened by all this.

My mother started going to church with Aunt Camille. On those occasions, my father would stay home to look after me. This gave him a good excuse not to go, as he just didn't understand this new "religion." My father was a small man with a slight stoop in his back from years of sewing and altering clothes. His dream was to own his own men's clothing store with a tailor shop in the back. Now that he was supporting a sick son, he knew those dreams would never come true. He had no extra money but was a meticulous dresser. Sometimes customers would not return for their altered clothing and he was able to buy those items at a much reduced cost. It was a real point of pride for him. Other than this small pleasure, for him life was a big disappointment. My father was born somewhere in Italy around Naples. He served in the Italian army during WWI and somehow he ended up fighting for the American army. We were never told the complete story of his wartime adventures, however after the war he got on an American Army transport ship and made his way to New York. He settled in Newark, New Jersey and there he met my mother. Just like me, my father was without hope and resigned to the fact that his dreams would never come true.

My mother started to go to church several times each week. I could tell there was a difference in her. She talked about Jesus more and more and she would read the Bible all the time. One Wednesday night when she got home from church, she came into the living room and she was glowing.

"Hi, Ma, you look real happy tonight, how was church?" I asked.

"Sonny," she began, "I've accepted Jesus Christ as my Lord and Savior." She beamed.

"What do you mean?" I asked.

"At the end of the service the pastor invited anyone who would, to come down to the altar and pray to receive Jesus. He said that if we did that, Jesus would come and make his home inside of us and we would be saved. Sonny, I went to the altar, I asked Jesus to forgive me for my sins and come into my heart and He did. I am born again and saved, my sins have been forgiven. I have never felt this way, this free." She explained.

Not knowing how to respond I said, "Gee, that's great Ma." I had heard my Aunt Camille talk like this for a few years now but I just didn't understand it all.

"Sonny, you can have this too. You can be free even though you think you are a prisoner in your own body, you can be free!" She urged.

"I don't know Ma. If God wanted me to be free, why did he let this happen to me?" I asked.

"The Bible says, 'And we know that in all things God works for the good of those who love Him, who have been called according to His purpose,'" she said.

"I'm not ready for this. I'll have to think about it." I replied.

"Sonny, I spoke to some of the Elders at church and one of them has a van. He said he could pick us up Sunday morning and they would carry us to church. How does that sound?" She asked.

I replied, "Let me think about this. It's so embarrassing to be carried around like that and in front of so many people."

My mother responded, "There is a story in the Bible about a group of men who carried their friend on a mat to see Jesus. This man was paralyzed. But these men had faith. Jesus was in his house at the time teaching the Gospel. There was such a crowd in and outside of the house that it was impossible to get to Jesus. The men would not give up. They carried their friend, who was still on his mat, up to the roof of Jesus' house. They dug a hole in the roof and then lowered their friend down to Jesus. Jesus forgave the paralyzed man for his sins and then healed him."

"Are you saying if I go to church, Jesus will heal me, come on now." I said with a little sarcasm.

"Sonny, I don't know what will happen. I do know that Jesus is real and alive and will help you. Please go next Sunday." She pleaded.

Well, I didn't know what to say. She's been so good to me and it seemed so important to her, that I agreed to go to church on the next Sunday. So what if I'm a little embarrassed. It might be good to get out of the house. She was so excited and said she would make arrangements with the church elders. She asked me to pray with her and I said that it would be ok. She sat next to my wheelchair and asked God to open my heart to His calling and to draw me to His son Jesus. When she was through praying, she said glory to God and Amen. I said Amen as well just to make her feel good.

CHAPTER 4

THE WATERING

The rest of the week I was a little nervous about going to church. Maybe it was my pride, the little of that I had left, but a voice inside of me kept trying to discourage me from going to the Sunday Service.

"Why put yourself through this embarrassment? You know, everyone in church will be staring at you, the cripple. They will pity you. Is that what you want?" This internal voice argued against my going to church. Over and over these thoughts ran through my mind.

Next, that inner voice reminded me that God let this happen to me. The inner voice quoted the same scripture that my mother mentioned, "And we know that in all things God works for the good of those who love Him, who have been called according to His purpose." "Yeah right, do you call being stricken with MS, "good", what possible good has this done you? You've lost everything. If God really loved you; you would not be in this situation." The voice harassed me mercilessly.

These inner arguments continued and grew in intensity as Sunday slowly but surely approached. That Saturday night I told my mother, "Ma, I don't think I am gonna go to church tomorrow. I really don't feel up to it. Maybe some other time, ok."

My mother would not have any of that. She replied, "Sonny, no, I can't accept that. You are going to go to church tomorrow no matter what. Ben McGraw and his brother Harold will be here with their van around 9:30 tomorrow morning and we'll be ready and waiting. I feel very strongly in my spirit that you are supposed to go, that you need to go to church tomorrow." She patted my head to comfort me and said, "Sonny, trust me, you'll be glad that you went. I just know that you will."

She asked me to pray about church in the morning. I agreed and I did pray, but it still didn't ease my anxiety about going. However, because of my mother's determination, I resolved in my mind that I would indeed go to church. When I did, that inner voice in my mind became silent.

That night I didn't sleep very well. I rationalized to myself that by this time tomorrow all this church stuff will be over. I won't have to go again and will be able to tell my mother that at least I tried it but church just was not for me.

Sunday morning came and my mother and father helped me get ready to leave the apartment and prepare to go to church. I hadn't been to church in years and never to a church that wasn't Catholic. So there I was sitting in my wheelchair waiting for the McGraw brothers to come for me. I was really dreading this. The door bell rang and in came these two big black men. The New Albany Church of God was one of the few churches in Albany with a mixed congregation. I had always gotten along well with the blacks, so that was not a problem for me.

"Good morning sister Mary and this must be your son Frank," said Ben, the older of the two men. "Brother Frank, we are so happy that you will be worshipping the Lord with us today. I just know you will receive a blessing," Ben promised.

There was a real sweetness about Ben and his brother Harold and I started to think that maybe this church thing wasn't going to be so terrible after all. These two men were part of the church's music ministry team. The two brothers plus two other church members played the music at the services and called themselves "The Abundant Life Quartet."

The New Albany Church of God held their services in the old Freihofer Bakery building on Spruce Street in Albany. The church purchased the building the year before and it was perfect for their worship services. What used to be a warehouse area was now the sanctuary that could easily hold up to 500 people. Folding chairs set up in straight lines faced the altar which consisted of a raised wooden platform with a simple podium that Ben and some of the other men constructed. Behind the altar, suspended from the steel girders that supported the ceiling, there was a rough hewn wooden cross. I was surprised to see that unlike the crosses in a Catholic church, there was no statue of Jesus. I would later find out that the empty cross emphasized Jesus resurrection. The sanctuary still had that industrial feel and was in stark contrast to the ornate Catholic Churches that I had grown up in.

The worship service began at 10:15 and we arrived at 10:00. The old Freihofer's employee parking lot provided ample parking for those attending the services. Ben and his brother were quite strong and had no trouble lifting me in and out of the van in my chair. They wheeled me into the vestibule and before we even entered the sanctuary, I was surrounded by church members wanting to introduce themselves and to tell me how happy they were that I came to the service. I was starting to feel comfortable and actually glad that I decided to come. They wheeled me to the end of an aisle as the sanctuary quickly filled. An organist played softly as we prepared to worship.

Ben McGraw opened the service with a prayer. He then welcomed everyone and introduced me. "We have a very special guest here with us today," he began, "Sister Mary Angelo's son Frank is with us for the first time. Please be sure to make him feel right at home." We sang several songs that I wasn't familiar with but I really enjoyed singing and then the pastor, a man named Brother Anthony, stepped up to the podium to deliver a message from the Book of Acts, the 2nd Chapter. As a boy in the Catholic Church I had heard about "The Book of The Acts of the Apostles" but I had never read it or even knew what it was about, so this was all very new to me. Brother Anthony told how the apostles were all together in this room in Jerusalem after Jesus' resurrection. Suddenly, they heard a sound of a violent wind and they saw tongues of fire that separated and came to rest on each of them. Brother Anthony explained that they were filled with the Holy Spirit. These people, who previously had been fearful and timid, were now emboldened and began to speak in languages that were unknown to them. Brother Anthony explained about speaking in "tongues," as a manifestation of the Holy Spirit. He said that we should all desire to pray in the Spirit this way and that it was a gift of the Spirit. He explained that we were all gifted differently as the Spirit saw fit.

In the Book of Acts, Peter, full of the Holy Spirit, began to preach to a crowd of several thousand who had gathered because they heard all the commotion stirred up by the apostles speaking in strange languages. Peter gave a convincing talk that Jesus was indeed the Messiah and the Lord. The people in the crowd were convicted of their sins and cut to the heart and they asked Peter and the other apostles, "Brothers, what shall we do?" Peter replied, "Repent and be baptized, every one of you, in the name of Jesus Christ for forgiveness of your sins. And you will receive the gift of the Holy Spirit."

Brother Anthony told us that salvation was God's gift to us. We cannot earn it because you can't earn a gift. God wants all of us to accept Jesus as our Lord and Savior and all we had to do is ask Jesus to come into our hearts and to forgive us for our sins and we will be saved. If we would do that, the Lord will live within us and if we surrender to the Holy Spirit, he will guide our lives. Brother Anthony invited all who wanted to accept Jesus in this way for the first time or anyone who wished to rededicate their lives to the Lord to come up to the altar. I felt a real tug on my heart to ask for help to get to the altar. My mother looked over at me encouraging me to do so. But I just couldn't do it. I wasn't ready or maybe I was too embarrassed to have someone wheel me to the front. At any rate I didn't go.

After the service, Brother Ben gave me a Bible. Ben suggested that I start by reading the Gospels, especially the Gospel of John. He said that was his favorite. Everyone came up to me to tell me how happy they were that I came and said to please come back. They all said that they would be praying for me.

The rest of that day all I could think about was Brother Anthony's sermon. I was very glad that I went to the service and now couldn't believe I had been so nervous about going in the first place. Maybe I should have gone up to the altar. I began reading the Gospel of John. In the 3rd Chapter, the 16th verse it says, "For God so loved the world that he gave his one and only son, that whoever believes in him shall not perish but have eternal life." It was just as Brother Anthony said, "Believe in Jesus, ask him to forgive you for your sins and invite him to be Lord of your life and you'll be saved." It was all so simple yet difficult at the same time. This message didn't come with a lot of rules and regulations. This message was a message of relationship.

That night I prayed to God that he would heal me and if he wanted me to accept Jesus, that he would give me the courage to do so. There would be a church service in a few days on Wednesday evening. The next morning I told my mother that I wanted to go with her and she was delighted. I continued to pray.

CHAPTER 5

ACCEPTING JESUS

Wednesday came and that inner voice started up again, "Do you really want to go to church and make a fool of yourself? What if your friends hear about this? I can just hear them now, "Did you hear about Sonny? He got sick and now he's one of those crazy holy rollers. Can you believe that?"

I told my mother that I changed my mind and would not be going with her that evening. But her reaction was the same as Sunday. "Sonny, no, I already made arrangements with Ben and Harold and they will be here at 6 tonight. Sorry, you've got to go."

Like clockwork, the two brothers were at our apartment at 6 o'clock. They told me how wonderful it was that I was going to join them for services and that I was sure to be blessed tonight. They heard that Brother Anthony had prepared a very special message.

When we arrived at church, I was amazed to find the place was packed. There were at least as many people at church on Wednesday night as had been there on Sunday. I was very impressed with how committed they were to the Lord. Growing up, going to Mass was more of an obligation, or at least it was for me. I always tried to get to an early Mass because they were short and you could get it "out of the way." God forbid if you got stuck going to a high Mass that lasted over an hour. That was torture and it seemed as if those masses would never be over. Church back then was an obligation, something you just had to do, not something you wanted to do. Now, I'm sure that many people didn't feel the same way about that but most of the people I knew certainly did.

Just like on Sunday, the people couldn't have been more welcoming, more loving. They genuinely seemed happy that I came to the service. I didn't feel at all out of place sitting there in my wheelchair. My Aunt Camille brought a friend with her to the service. "Sonny, I want you to meet my friend Judy Tortelli. This is her first visit to our church." Camille explained. Judy was about my age and she seemed very nervous and a little out of place.

"Hi Judy, don't worry, this is only my second time. You'll find everyone is so warm and loving. In no time, you'll feel at home." I said, trying to encourage her. She smiled at me. I think my words helped her, knowing that she wasn't the only newcomer.

Once again the service started with singing a few worship songs. At this point, my voice was still strong enough to sing. Singing had been such an important part of my life but it had been a while since I felt like singing about anything. When we finished, Ben asked everyone to pass the peace of Christ to one another by greeting those around you. Several people came up to me and said they heard me sing and commented on how beautiful my voice was. One person suggested that some Sunday I should sing a solo. That encouragement really lifted my spirits.

Brother Anthony began his sermon by telling us that he was going to preach a message from the Book of Romans and the Book of Luke. The message would be about two roads, the Romans Road to Salvation and the Road to Emmaus. I had my Bible; the one Ben gave me on Sunday, and was glad that I did because Brother Anthony asked us to open our Bibles to Romans. The Bible was still new to me, so my mother quietly helped me find Romans so as not to embarrass me.

The pastor began by saying there were five stops on the Romans Road to Salvation. First he read, "For all have sinned, and come short of the glory of God." He explained that we were all sinners and there is no one who is innocent.

The second stop on the road, he explained, dealt with the "consequences" of sin. "For the wages of sin is death." The punishment that we have earned due to our sins is death. Not just physical death but eternal death!

Next came the good news, "But the gift of God is eternal life through Jesus Christ our Lord." And, "God demonstrates His own love toward us, in that while we were still sinners, Christ died for us." Brother Anthony started to get very excited and emotional at this point. He had to stop for a moment and compose himself and several people began to praise God. They were praising God, lifting their hands and several of them were speaking in a strange language that I found out later was called "tongues." This is what we used to mock. Even some of my family members, my uncle Peter in particular, would joke about, "those holy rollers." However, seeing it in person and seeing the faith and the sincerity, I found it something to envy not to mock. The pastor continued, "People, just think about it, Jesus died for us. He died for you and me! He paid the price for our sins and Jesus' resurrection proves that God the Father accepted Jesus the Son's death as payment for our sins."

The fourth stop on the Romans Road to Salvation is what we need to do, "that if you confess with your mouth Jesus is Lord, and believe in your heart that God raised Him from the dead, you will be saved." The pastor explained Jesus' death on the cross paid the penalty for our sins. All we have to do is believe in Jesus and if we do we will be saved. Our salvation, the forgiveness of our sins, is available to anyone who will trust in Jesus as their Lord and Savior.

The final stop on the Romans Road is the result of salvation. "Therefore, since we have been justified through faith, we have peace with God through our Lord Jesus Christ." Because of Jesus, we can have a relationship and peace with God. Brother Anthony read Romans 8:1, "Therefore, there is now no condemnation for those who are in Christ Jesus." For a good Catholic boy like me this was amazing news. Because of Jesus' death for us, we will never be condemned for our sins. Brother Anthony said that we have this promise from God, "For I am convinced that neither death nor life, neither angels nor demons, neither the present nor the future, nor any powers, neither height nor depth, nor anything else in all creation, will be able to separate us from the love of God that is in Christ Jesus our Lord."

The church was stirred by the pastor's words. Shouts of "Praise God!" and "Amen!" filled the sanctuary. Brother Anthony went on to talk about two travelers on the Road to Emmaus. These two men were disciples of Jesus. They had left Jerusalem after Jesus had been crucified and were heading to the small town called Emmaus. They were dejected and upset because their Lord was gone, or so they thought. Then Jesus came up to them and began walking with them but the Bible says "they were kept from recognizing Him." Jesus asked them what was wrong because they were obviously upset. They explained that Jesus of Nazareth, a prophet of great power and deeds, was crucified by the chief priests and Roman officials. They said they were sad because they had hoped that he was going to be the one who redeemed Israel. They told their new companion that some of their women claimed that Jesus' tomb was empty and that they had an encounter with angels who claimed Jesus was alive. They said that some of their companions had gone to the tomb and indeed the tomb was empty!

The two men were confused and depressed by all of this. They just didn't understand. But Jesus said to them, "How foolish you are, and how slow of heart to believe all that the prophets have spoken! Did not the Christ have to suffer these things and then enter His glory?" The pastor quoted the Bible, "And beginning with Moses and all the Prophets, he explained to them what was said in all the Scriptures concerning himself." As they approached Emmaus, Jesus acted as if he were going farther but the two travelers urged him to stay with them as it was late in the day. So Jesus did. Brother Anthony interjected, "If you ask Jesus to stay with you, he always will. He'll never leave you, he said so. Do you believe that?" The whole church shouted a resounding, "Amen!"

Jesus and the two travelers sat down to eat and Jesus took bread, gave thanks, broke it and began to give it to them. The two travelers' eyes were opened and at that point they recognized Jesus and he disappeared from their sight.

"Folks," Brother Anthony said, "Jesus died for your sins, and three days later he defeated death and rose from the dead. He is alive but you have to believe. Open your eyes and accept him tonight! After Jesus disappeared from their sight, the two travelers asked each other. 'Were not our hearts burning within us while he talked with us on the road and opened the Scriptures to us?' Why couldn't they recognize Jesus before? Faith comes from hearing the message and the message is heard through the word of Christ! When Jesus opened the Scriptures to them, they were shot through with faith!"

Brother Anthony gave the altar call, "Anyone who wants to accept Jesus as their Lord and Savior, come down the "Road to Salvation" up to this altar right now. Get on the right side of the Walls of Salvation. Don't be afraid, Jesus says, 'Do not be afraid, I will always be with you and will never leave you!"

My heart was burning! If I was still able to use my legs, I would have run up to that altar. Looking over to my mother, I saw tears were streaming from her eyes and I whispered for her to wheel me up to the altar.

By the time I reached the altar I was sobbing. Brother Anthony said, "Frank, are you ready to accept Jesus as your Lord and Savior?" I said, "Yes, sir." He laid his hands on my shoulders and asked me to say this prayer, "Lord God, I know that I am a sinner and deserving of punishment. But Jesus Christ took the punishment that I deserve, so that through faith in him I could be forgiven. I am truly sorry, and now I turn away from my past sinful life to follow you. Please forgive me. Please help me not to return to my life of sin. I believe that your son, Jesus Christ, died for my sins, was resurrected from the dead, is alive and hears my prayer. I ask Jesus to become the Lord of my life and to rule and reign in my heart from this day forward. Please send your Holy Spirit to enable me to obey you and to do your will for the rest of my life. In Jesus' name I pray, Amen."

As I finished saying that prayer, joy filled my heart. It didn't matter that I was there sitting in a wheelchair. The only thing that mattered was Jesus! The shouts of praise and the hand clapping from the congregation was so loud, it felt as though the building shook.

I was a new creation. The old had gone, the new had come! The date, May 20, 1955 was my new birthday, the day I gave my life to the Lord.

Several people including Brother Anthony came to our house the next Sunday to celebrate my big day. My mother made her wonderful lasagna the night before and had plenty for everyone. After lunch Brother Anthony sat down next to me and opened his Bible to Matthew 3:13-17 and read:

> Then Jesus came from Galilee to the Jordan to be baptized by John. But John tried to deter him, saying, "I need to be baptized by you, and do you come to me?"

> Jesus replied, "Let it be so now; it is proper for us to do this to fulfill all righteousness." Then John consented.

> As soon as Jesus was baptized, he went up out of the water. At that moment heaven was opened, and he saw the Spirit of God descending like a dove and lighting on him. And a voice from heaven said, "This is my Son, whom I love; with him I am well pleased."

"Frank, now that you have accepted Jesus as your Lord and Savior, I think you should follow his example and be baptized," said Brother Anthony.

I replied, "I want to be obedient to the Lord but I'm in this wheelchair. I've heard my mother and Aunt Camille talk about baptism and being completely submerged under water. We can't put my chair under the water?"

"Frank, we won't have to. Praise God, we've had several people come to the Lord this month. The elders and I have been talking about having a special church service out at Miracle Lake in a couple of weeks. The service will include baptisms in the lake. It would be easy to put you on a stretcher and then some of the men could carry you into the water. What do you think about that?" Brother Anthony asked me.

I must admit, I was hesitant, that whole making a spectacle of myself thing again. But, how could I refuse the Lord. If Jesus, the Son of God, was baptized to show us the way, how could I not follow him? I said to Brother Anthony, "Yes, will you make the arrangements for the stretcher?" He said he would.

Two weeks later, I and several other Christian brothers and sisters waited by the shoreline of Miracle Lake. One of the church members was a high school football coach and he provided a stretcher that the team always brought to their games in case a player became injured. The elders helped me out of my wheelchair and onto the stretcher. Then we waded into the lake where Brother Anthony stood waiting waist deep in the water.

"Are you ready, Brother Frank?" He asked, as he smiled broadly at me. I nodded that I was and held my nose preparing to go under the water. Brother Anthony placed his right hand on my forehead and raised his other hand to the Lord and prayed, "Brother Frank, I baptize thee in the name of the Father and of the Son and of the Holy Spirit," and with that the elders slowly began to lower me into Miracle Lake until I was completely buried by the water.

I was only immersed in the water for a second or two but something happened as they raised me back above the water. A brilliant light flashed across my mind and the Lord spoke to me saying, "Trust me, you will never be out of my sight." As I came up out of the water, I received what I would later find out was the "Baptism of the Holy Spirit" and began speaking in tongues. I didn't understand what I was saying but Brother Anthony, who has the gift of interpreting tongues, told me and the congregation that I said, "Trust in the Lord always!"

As with so many of my early Christian experiences, I had gone into this with fearful anticipation but came out of it with joyful exuberance. I guess the lesson I was learning was to trust God and follow the leading of his Holy Spirit. You will never go wrong if you do.

CHAPER 6

MY NEW LIFE

After accepting Jesus as my Lord and Savior, my primary interest was to get to know him better. I spent hours each day reading the Bible. There was so much to learn. It was all new and very exciting. With every verse there was another discovery and with every day I grew closer to him.

Ben suggested that I start by reading the Gospels especially the Gospel of John. In the fifteenth Chapter and fifteenth verse, Jesus tells His disciples, "I no longer call you servants, because a servant does not know his master's business. Instead, I have called you friends, for everything that I learned from my Father I have made known to you." To think that Jesus would consider me his friend was too wonderful. I was bound by my wheelchair but I was soaring like an eagle.

Being in love with the Lord was something so great I couldn't keep it to myself. Brother Anthony came to see me a couple of weeks after I gave my life to the Lord. He wanted to find out how I was doing and to see if I had any questions about my new faith that he could answer. Brother Anthony was an Italian in his mid fifties with a full head of hair that was once black but now peppered with gray. He was a handsome man, small in stature but a very powerful presence. Like most of the congregation at the New Albany Church of God, he had once been a Catholic. In fact, he had graduated from the seminary. Because he questioned some points of the Catholic doctrine, he was not allowed to take his final vows and be ordained. Rather than recant his position on what we must do to be saved and complete the required penance, Brother Anthony left the Church. Over the years, he studied the Bible extensively and was active in a large Pentecostal Church in Buffalo, where he taught Sunday school and became an assistant pastor. Five years ago, he felt a strong leading of the Lord to come to Albany to start a church.

"Brother Frank," he asked, "How have your first few weeks been as a new creation in the Lord?"

I told him about my hunger for the Lord, that I couldn't read enough of the Bible and more than anything I wanted to share Jesus with everyone. I asked him, "I'm bound by this chair. What can I do to serve the Lord?"

Without any hesitation he answered, "Brother Frank, as pastor, I am called upon to visit hospitals and nursing homes several times each week. So many people who are sick and hurting need a friend. They need encouragement and they need to meet Jesus. You understand what it is to be sick and hurt and you would be perfect to bring the good news of our Lord Jesus to them."

I replied, "But I can't get up, walk downstairs to the bus stop and go to Albany Medical Center to talk to someone."

"Yes, that's true, but you can write a letter. I can't tell you how much it means to those confined to their hospital beds to receive a card or letter; so many of them have no one who cares. But you and I know that Jesus cares. You could write letters and share your story introducing them to Jesus. Jesus taught that ministering to the least of his children is the same as ministering to him." Brother Anthony explained.

"But I've only been with the Lord a few weeks. Shouldn't I wait awhile and learn more. I mean you've been studying for decades. Witnessing must come easy to you?" I questioned.

"Frank, it will not be you witnessing but the Holy Spirit. You know Brother Ben. What a wonderful brother in Christ he is. He is a humble man. He doesn't have a high school diploma. He's never been to seminary but he is one of the most effective witnesses for Christ that I know. Ben goes into the Albany County jail every week to hand out Bibles and witnesses to the men who are locked up. He has led many to the Lord. Several of those men are now members of our church. I recall someone asking Ben about his preparation before he went to speak at one of the services he holds at the jail. They asked him how much time did it take him to prepare a message. He said five minutes. They were amazed as his sermons often last thirty minutes or more. He explained that the Gospel message was simple. He just tells them what Jesus means to him. Frank, you can do that, can't you?" Brother Anthony concluded.

I agreed with Brother Anthony that with the Holy Spirit as my guide I could do that. He said that he would provide me with the names of the patients in the various facilities he visits each week. He would also tell me, as best as he could, the nature of their illness. I could write letters and bring them to him at the Sunday or Wednesday night services. When Brother Anthony went on his visits, he would deliver the letters and tell them a little bit about me.

The next Sunday at church, Brother Anthony, true to his word handed me a sheet of paper with information about several patients including something about their ailments and a little bit about their history. I could hardly wait to get home and start writing to them about Jesus. I assured Brother Anthony that I would have the letters ready for him by Wednesday evening service.

In the beginning of this letter writing ministry, I was still able to hold a pen and write. My penmanship was always very good and quite legible. From then on, if someone asked what I wanted for my birthday or Christmas, I would always say, "stationery."

Keeping in mind Brother Anthony's example of Ben McGraw's jailhouse ministry, I kept the message simple. I just wrote about how much Jesus loves us, how he will never leave us or forsake us. I wrote to them that no matter how bad things became, not to give up because our Lord understands suffering.

I continued to study the Bible and about a month after I accepted the Lord, I began to be troubled by the question of healing. The Gospels detail Jesus earthly ministry and a big part of his ministry was healing. Some of the people I had written to wrote back to me asking about healing. They said that they had prayed many times to be healed but God had not answered their prayers. One Sunday at church I asked Brother Anthony about this. He said that he believed in spiritual healing and in fact had personally witnessed some miraculous healings. I told him that I read in the Book of James, "Is any one sick? He should call the elders of the church to pray over him and anoint him with oil in the name of the Lord. And the prayer offered in faith will make the sick person well."

Brother Anthony said that he would gather several of the elders after the service and we would go to one of the classrooms and pray for my healing. I was so excited by this. I knew God would heal me just as he had healed so many in the Bible. My faith was soaring. After the service my mother wheeled me back to one of the Sunday school classrooms. Brother Anthony, Ben and Harold McGraw and two other elders were waiting for me. Ben held a small bottle of oil. Brother Anthony said, "Brother Frank, do you believe Jesus can heal you?"

I replied, "Yes sir, I do."

The elders all laid hands on me. Brother Ben anointed my forehead with oil and the elders prayed for me. For thirty minutes they pleaded with the Lord to make me whole and to restore my health. Despite my faith, I didn't feel any difference in my body. Brother Anthony told me not to be discouraged, "everything happens according to God's timing not ours," he said. On the next two Sundays the elders and Brother Anthony laid hands on me, anointed me with oil and pleaded with the Lord to take this MS from me. But again there was no change in my condition. They concluded that at this time it was not God's will that I should receive a healing.

I was very discouraged. The enemy seizing the opportunity because of my weakness and discouragement began to attack me. For several days an inner voice kept trying to persuade me that this relationship with Jesus was all a bunch of hooey. "Just give up and die," the voice kept repeating. In addition to that, strange things began to happen in our apartment. For three nights in a row, I was awakened by a lamp falling on the floor. There was no reason for the lamp to be knocked over but it just happened. Another night we apparently had an electrical short in our doorbell. The doorbell would not stop ringing, at three o'clock in the morning! The next night the TV set turned on by itself. All of this happened in one week.

My mother told her sister, Camille, about these strange things and also about my discouragement. Aunt Camille was very strong in the Lord. She had what Brother Anthony called the gift of prophecy and had the ability to discern spirits. She came over to the house and sat down with my mother and me. We held hands and prayed for wisdom. Camille began praying in tongues. She told us that indeed the enemy was harassing us. Demons had been dispatched to try to scare us and disrupt my walk with the Lord. Camille said, "Frank, the enemy fears you and the potential you have as a servant of Jesus, so be strong and do not be afraid." Camille said she had received a word of knowledge from the Lord concerning my healing. "Frank, the Lord says that you should read 2 Corinthians Chapter 12."

2 Corinthians Chapter 12 is about Paul's thorn in his flesh. Paul wrote, "To keep me from becoming conceited because of these surpassingly great revelations, there was given me a thorn in my flesh, a messenger of Satan, to torment me. Three times I pleaded with the Lord to take it away from me. But He (Jesus) said to me, 'My grace is sufficient for you, for my power is made perfect in weakness.'

Therefore I will boast all the more gladly about my weaknesses, so that Christ's power may rest on me. That is why, for Christ's sake, I delight in weaknesses, in insults, in hardships, in persecutions, in difficulties. For when I am weak, then I am strong."

It was clear, at least for now, that the Lord would not heal me but he would strengthen me. At least now I knew. I would go on trusting him that when I am weak, then I am strong. I was now able to respond to those I was ministering to that sometimes the grace of our Lord Jesus Christ will have to suffice and during those times his grace will be sufficient, we have his promise.

Armed with this knowledge and the power of the Holy Spirit, we prayed that the Lord would rebuke the enemy and not allow him to harass us. The attacks stopped immediately and we slept well at night from then on. Brother Anthony was a strong believer in always putting on the Armor of God the first thing every morning. He told Camille, "The enemy is persistent and we should be as well." He found this prayer that was an adaptation of Ephesians 6:10–20. He recommended that Camille make this prayer part of her morning worship. After this bout with the enemy my mother and I did the same. Here is the Spiritual Warfare Prayer:

> I am strong in You Lord, and in the power of your might. I put on the whole armor of God and do stand against the plans of the devil. In the name of Jesus, I bind Satan and the principalities, the powers, the rulers of the darkness of this world. I bind and cast down spiritual wickedness in high places and render them harmless and ineffective against me and my loved ones. I resist you devil, in the name of Jesus and I stand my ground.

> I have the Belt of Truth buckled around my waist – the Truth of God that sets me free! I have on the Breastplate of Righteousness that covers my body, my heart and vital organs and shows me I am in right standing with my God! My feet are shod with the Preparation of the Gospel of Peace, and I take those feet and tread on serpents and scorpions, for I have been given authority over all your power. I take the Helmet of Salvation and cover my head securely, for I have the Mind of Christ. The only spirit I will follow is the Spirit

of the Living God that lives inside me and speaks to me from within.

I take the Shield of Faith and quench every arrow you throw at me, devil! I take the Sword of the Spirit, which is the Word of God, and pierce through your wicked plans, for it is written, all I have to do is submit myself to God, and tell you to flee, and you have to go…so GO, in the name of Jesus!

I place the Blood of Jesus over me, my family, my home, my ministry, my possessions, all that you have given me and all of it belongs to God and I serve notice that your power is broken, devil, over me and mine, in Jesus name.

Thank you Father, please send people my way to minister to today. Amen

The next day I was alone in my room and praying that the Holy Spirit would indeed use me as Camille had prophesized that he would. I had the covers pulled over my head as I prayed. Suddenly, I felt consumed by the fire of the Holy Spirit and began speaking in tongues. This was the first of many times that I would experience what I would describe as a refilling of the Holy Spirit. Not only was I praying in tongues but for the first time I understood what I was praying. I found out later that this was called the Gift of Interpretation. The Holy Spirit was praying through me and telling me that, "Indeed, my power is made perfect in your weakness, be strong and very courageous." Amen and Amen!

CHAPTER 7

MINISTRY

It was a Tuesday afternoon. I was sitting in my room reading my Bible. The door bell rang and my mother welcomed Ben McGraw. "Brother Frank, how are you feeling today?" He said with a beaming smile, as he walked in the room and sat down on the couch.

"Ben, it's so good to see you. Just stopping by for a visit?" I asked.

"Frank, I have a favor to ask. Several of our church members have commented to me about what a fine singing voice you have. I was wondering. Would you consider singing a solo this Sunday at church?" He inquired.

He took me by surprise. I hadn't thought about singing in front of a group in awhile let alone in church. But the Holy Spirit wouldn't let me off the hook and almost without thinking, I heard myself saying, "Yes."

After talking it over and at Ben's urging we decided to do "It is Well with My Soul." We worked it out that we would rehearse the song after the Wednesday night service. Ben, anticipating that I would agree, brought a song book, in case I didn't know the song. Indeed, I was not familiar with it but after reading the lyrics and practicing on my own that night, it became my favorite song.

My excitement grew as Wednesday night approached. I couldn't wait until I got to rehearse with the group. The Abundant Life Quartet was amazing and Ben was such a gifted piano player. The first time we rehearsed the song, I was thrilled. Ben and the guys went on and on about what a blessing this would be for the church.

The days until Sunday were filled with anticipation. When the moment arrived and Brother Anthony introduced me, I had to calm myself down. I was so excited to once again have the opportunity to sing in public. It could not have gone better. The church gave me a standing ovation. Everyone came up to me after the service to tell me what a blessing they received and how talented I was. I thought to myself, I may be in this wheel chair but I was back.

On the way home, I was feeling pretty good about myself when suddenly this wave of guilt swept over me. Was I singing to glorify the Lord or to glorify myself? Pride is so subtle. Immediately, I asked the Lord to forgive me. The Lord said to "be holy, because I am holy." Becoming holy is a process and I still had a long way to go. This was a lesson I needed to bring into all areas of my life especially to ministry. It should be a joy to bless others and to somehow bring glory to God.

With that lesson in mind, it was such a joy to correspond with so many people who, like me, faced physical challenges each day. Several told me that because of my letters and Brother Anthony's help, they had accepted Jesus as their Lord and Savior. Brother Anthony told me we made a great team. My letters planted a seed and he reaped the harvest for the glory of God.

Because of my letters, several patients at the Albany County Convalescent Home asked Brother Anthony if it were possible for me to come for a visit and perhaps give a talk in the chapel. He asked me if I was up for this and if so, he would arrange for a couple of the men to transport me. At first I was hesitant however this was an opportunity I couldn't pass up. Besides, I really wanted to finally meet the people at the county home.

The next Thursday was the day Brother Anthony usually visited the county home and held a service. The McGraw brothers arrived to take me. They always had a smile on their face and tried to be a blessing to everyone they came in contact with. The county home was a very sad and dreary place, in fact, shabby was the best word to describe it. People who had little or no money and no one capable or willing to care for them, came to the home to die. It was a very depressing place and all the more reason that we needed to be there. Jesus taught in the Gospel of Matthew, "For I was hungry and you gave me something to eat, I was thirsty and you gave me something to drink, I was a stranger and you invited me in, I was sick and you looked after me, I was in prison and you came to visit me. I tell you the truth, whatever you did for one of the least of these brothers of mine, you did for me." This was an opportunity to bless the Lord by helping the least of his brothers. I rejoiced that I could do this. I prayed that I would not end up here at the Albany County Convalescent Home and my heart went out to those who did.

It was almost Thanksgiving and after praying about what I should talk about during the chapel service, I felt led by the Spirit to talk about being thankful. The chapel was full as maybe thirty-five residents were wheeled in. A few came in with the aid of a walker. I began my message talking about how Jesus healed ten men who had leprosy. Jesus was traveling along the border between Samaria and Galilee when he met these men on the road. Those with leprosy always kept their distance so they called out to him shouting, "Jesus, Master, have pity on us!" Jesus said to them. "Go, show yourselves to the priests." As they went they were healed. But only one of them, when he saw he was healed, came back, shouting praises to God. He fell at Jesus feet and thanked him and this man was a Samaritan. Samaritans were people of mixed race, half Jewish and half Assyrian, and they were looked down upon by the Jews. Jesus asked him where the other nine were. "Was no one found to return and give praise to God except this foreigner? Rise and go; your faith has made you well." How often do we forget to give God thanks? Even though, our very breath depends on him.

Then I told them about this lady named Corrie ten Boom. I read an article about Miss ten Boom and her faith impressed me so much. She was a Dutch Christian and a Holocaust survivor. She was imprisoned because she helped many Jews escape the Nazis. After suffering extreme cruelty at the hands of the SS, she and her sister Betsie were sent to a concentration camp in Ravensbruck. The conditions at the camp were deplorable. They had no heat and very little food and were forced to perform strenuous manual labor, and Corrie was 50 years old at the time. They slept on straw mattresses that were filled with choking dust and swarming with fleas. Bibles were outlawed by the Nazis, however Corrie smuggled a copy of the four Gospels into the barracks. She held Bible studies and because of the fleas, the prison guards never checked inside the barracks. This allowed Corrie and her sister to teach the word of God without fear of reprisals from the Nazis. Corrie and Betsie thanked God for those awful fleas because it allowed them to preach the word of God! God was faithful to Corrie. Due to an "administrative error," she was released from the concentration camp. This was no error in her paperwork rather the hand of God was with her. She was given back her possessions that had been confiscated and sent back home to Holland. A week later the Germans executed all the women at Ravensbruck who were Corrie's age or older. I concluded my talk by reminding those in the chapel that we should be inspired by Corrie and thank God for all things, even the things in our life that cause us grief and pain can be used for his glory. "Let's not be like those nine lepers who did not return to thank Jesus, let's be like Corrie." I said.

My reception in chapel was wonderful. Many thanked me for coming and told me that my words were a blessing and comfort to them. It was great to personally meet the people with whom I had been corresponding for six months. As Brother Anthony was wheeling me out, a small, frail little woman who was wheelchair bound stopped us. Her name was Eva Grantland and she was eighty-eight years old. She had a stroke last year and could not move the left side of her body. The left side of her face was drooping and that made it difficult for her to speak. Her left arm was in a sling to keep it from shaking due to tremors. She was all alone. Her husband had passed away ten years ago and her only child, a son, died in the war.

Mrs. Grantland said to me, "Frank, it did my heart good to meet you. Whatever happens to you, no matter how bad things get, just remember that someday you and I will get brand new strong healthy bodies. Someday, you and I will run and jump again. Don't you forget that and never stop trusting God. Don't give up." I was there to encourage them and here she was, blessing me.

I never forgot Mrs. Grantland or the advice she gave me. Two months later she went to be with the Lord. I am convinced that somewhere up in heaven she indeed is walking and running and being a blessing.

One Sunday after church my mother cooked her wonderful lasagna and invited several family members over. It was one of the few times that all three of my sons were with us. My Uncle Peter and his family were also there. Peter had not yet come to the Lord. After the meal, Peter started suggesting that perhaps my illness was all in my mind and that if I would just try to stand up, I probably would be able to walk. The room became completely silent and everyone looked over at me to see what I would do, even my mother looked at me, as if she believed that if I determined in my mind to do so, I could indeed get out of my wheelchair and walk. My three sons all started to encourage me, hoping that perhaps they would get their healthy strong dad back. "Please try Dad, you can do it!" My youngest son Ricardo urged. Holding the arms of the chair as tightly as I could, I pushed with all the strength that remained in my arms and by sheer force of will was able to stand about three quarters of the way straight. It was too much for me and I ended up falling on the floor. Embarrassed by my failure, I looked at the disappointed faces of my sons. At least I tried. That was the last time I ever attempted to stand.

Gradually the strength in my voice began to weaken. Dr. Macumber had warned me this might happen. I could no longer use my voice to sing. This had been an important part of my life. It was part of who I was. But it was also a point of pride. With the help of the Holy Spirit, I accepted losing my voice as one more way God was breaking me down, molding me for his use. I had to trust him. He is the gardener and he decides just how to prune the branches. My eyesight was fine most days but there were days when all I could see was movement in a haze. Thanks to Jesus, my moods were under control. I no longer lost my temper and decided that I would thank God for each day he gave me. From 1955 to 1960 I went from needing a cane to requiring a wheelchair to becoming bedridden. Life was difficult. However, looking back I cannot imagine my life without Jesus. He was my sustainer.

When I began my letter writing ministry, I would carefully write letters on stationary. When it became too difficult to hold a pen, the church bought me a small typewriter. Although it took some time, I was able to peck out my letters on the typewriter. Eventually, my fingers lost their strength and even pecking on the keys was too difficult. My mother had a pet parakeet. There was a toy parakeet inside the bird cage that kept the little bird company. The toy bird was shaped in such a way that it was easy for me to grasp. My mother wrapped the toy with adhesive tape to improve the grip. Using the toy bird, I was again able to hit the typewriter keys with sufficient force to type a letter. It would sometimes take over an hour just to type one brief letter. However, with God's help I persisted. This worked for about 6 months, then the strength in my arms began to fail and I could no longer lift them.

Unable to write or type, I was still determined to continue my letter writing ministry. Led by the Holy Spirit, I determined that anyone who came to visit me would become my writing instrument that day. I asked my visitors if they would do me a favor. Naturally, they always said yes. I must say, that more than one person seemed a bit dismayed when I told them the favor was to write a letter for me as I dictated to them. Nevertheless, this was a wonderful ministry tool. Not only was I witnessing to the recipient of the letter but the person writing the letter was also hearing the word of God. God certainly works in wonderful and amazing ways.

My letter writing ministry would continue until 1970. At that point, I could barely speak above a whisper and my health really deteriorated. However, Brother Anthony told me near the end of the ministry, that in fifteen years he estimated that I sent over 5,000 letters. He said that he knew many of my pen pals who accepted Jesus because of my faithful witness through these letters. In addition, many people improved their lives by quitting smoking. If I knew that the person I was writing to was a smoker, I always urged them to quit and prayed for them to have the strength to do so. As a former smoker myself, I understood how difficult it was to quit but I also knew the benefits to your health. More than that, I believed that it was pleasing to God if we didn't pollute his temple with cigarette smoke.

The Lord had decided that his strength could be made more perfect in my weakness and indeed he was right.

CHAPTER 8

SISTER JUDY

It was about a month after I sang my solo when we had a visitor come to our apartment. I was quite surprised when Aunt Camille's friend Judy Tortelli walked into my room. She apologized for just dropping by but said she was in the neighborhood.

"Mrs. Angelo, I hope you don't mind me dropping by but I wanted to ask Frank if he might consider singing with me one Sunday. I was so moved when you sang "It is Well with My Soul" and I've been praying about this since then."

Judy had not missed a service at church since that Sunday when she first came with Aunt Camille. Two weeks later she walked up to the altar and accepted Jesus as her Lord and Savior. Camille privately shared with us a little bit of Judy's background. She first met Judy at the Miss Albany Diner where Judy was working as a waitress. Aunt Camille has such a heart for lonely and hurting people and as she said, "it was easy to see that Judy was in trouble and needed the Lord's help." She said that Judy was hiding a black eye by trying to conceal it with extra make-up. Apparently she was living with an abusive husband. Camille told us that Judy did her best to put up a brave front but it was obvious that behind her smile there was a lot of pain. Over several weeks of going to the diner, she and Judy became friends and eventually Judy began to confide in her. Camille had a friend working in the woman's ministry of the Salvation Army, and with their help, Judy found the strength to leave her abusive husband and was living at the Salvation Army's women's dormitory. She was indeed a new creation in Jesus and had an unquenchable thirst to know the Lord better and to serve him.

"Frank, there's a song that I heard down at the Salvation Army. It's called 'His Eye is on the Sparrow', do you know it?" Judy asked.

Many of the songs we sang at the New Albany Church of God were new to me. The songs I learned as a boy in the Catholic Church were primarily all in Latin. I replied, "No Judy, I don't know it, how does it go."

She began to sing so sweetly, "I sing because I'm happy, I sing because I'm free, for His eye is on the sparrow and I know He watches me."

It was a beautiful song based on scripture from Matthew 10:29 "Are not two sparrows sold for a penny? Yet not one of them will fall to the ground apart from the will of your Father. And even the very hairs of your head are all numbered. So don't be afraid; you are worth more than many sparrows." I thought to myself how much that verse meant to me and must have meant to Judy. What courage it took for her to leave her husband and to seek shelter in the arms of Jesus. And here I was in this wheelchair, my prognosis was bleak and I too had to take shelter in His loving arms.

"Judy, I love the song and I love the scripture verses that inspired it. It would be an honor to sing this with you." I said.

We agreed to practice after church Wednesday night and we worked everything out with Brother Anthony and Ben McGraw. Getting to know Judy was a delight. She had such a sweet spirit about her. When Sunday came along, we sang this beautiful song. But unlike the first time I sang in church, this song was to glorify Him. I believe everyone at the service was blessed by the important message of the song and more importantly that God was glorified. This was the last time I sang with the quartet in this capacity. My voice was growing too weak. But I will always look upon that Sunday, singing with Judy, as a special time, a time that I felt especially close to my Lord.

Judy and I grew to be great friends. She would come by the house from time to time to discuss the Lord. Sometimes she would sing to me. We would always pray. When we arrived at church, hers was the first face I would look for. On one of her visits to our apartment, I could tell something was troubling her. She seemed upset so I asked her, "Judy, what's on your mind?"

"Frank, I've been praying and thinking about joining the Salvation Army as a recruit. I've seen firsthand the work they do in the Lord's name and feel that the Holy Spirit is leading me to make that decision." She said.

I replied, "To be used by the Lord that way, I think that's wonderful."

"I think so too. But it means that I have to change churches. I'll have to be at the Salvation Army Services and won't be able to attend

The New Albany Church of God. I have grown to love the church and everyone there so much. And because of that, it makes me a little sad as well." She explained.

"Sometimes God asks us to do hard things. I know you love our church but surely you'll be able to visit once in awhile." I said, trying to comfort her. "Now tell me all about what you'll be doing."

Her eyes lit up as she began to tell me all that she would be doing to serve the Lord. "Right now I'm a recruit. I have a series of classes to complete and once I pass everything I will be presented to the Corps Pastoral Council for acceptance as a soldier. Hopefully, all will go well and during a Sunday Service I'll be sworn in as a soldier. I'll be a Salvationist and a soldier in God's army." She proudly explained.

"Judy, I'll pray for you every day. I know you'll be a blessing and bring glory to His name. I'm so proud of you." I said.

We saw Judy less and less over the next few months as her work and study with the Salvation Army increased. She did stop by one afternoon and invited us to attend the service at the Salvation Army the following Sunday. "Frank, I made it, praise God! I'm to be sworn in this Sunday. It would mean a lot to me if you could be there for the ceremony." She beamed.

We worked it out with Brother Anthony and borrowed the church van so that I could be present for Judy's swearing in. She looked so beautiful in her Salvation Army uniform with the blue epaulets. If I wasn't sick, I think I would have asked Judy to marry me. But as I told Judy, "sometimes God asks us to do hard things."

Judy went on to be a pillar for the poor and needy in Albany. She continued to study and was commissioned as an officer and was fully ordained in the Salvation Army. Officially she may have been Captain Judy Tortelli but she was known to the thousands over the years that were touched by her love and ministry simply as Sister Judy. Knowing her was one of the best things of my life.

CHAPTER 9

THREE MEN

Other than my family, I had two very close friends before I got sick. Tommy Phelan, my great friend and business partner and Johnny Canavi. These two had been my best friends since we were little boys. Tommy and Johnny were opposites bound together only by their relationship with me.

Tommy, Johnny and I were best friends since the 1st grade at P.S. 21 on Clinton Avenue. Tommy was always the biggest kid in school and as such was a great person to have as a best friend. Johnny on the other hand was always one of the smallest kids but he had all the guts in the world and a temper to match. Tommy was never one to get into a fight unless there was absolutely no other way but Johnny, he loved to fight. If you got into a fight with Johnny, you would just about have to kill him because he would keep on coming.

All three of us played baseball for Schuyler High School, although Johnny missed being on our championship team senior year after he dropped out of school. Tommy was the catcher, Johnny played second base and I was at first. One day after practice, when we were freshmen, word spread that Johnny was going to fight this senior, a guy by the name of Dennis Corcione. Apparently, Johnny had been messing with Dennis' girlfriend. Most of the team hung around after the coach left and sure enough Johnny and Dennis went at it. Dennis was at least 30 to 40 pounds heavier and was 3 years older than Johnny and really gave Johnny a beating. Eventually, we all stepped in and separated the guys to save Johnny's life. I believe Dennis would have continued to beat Johnny until he was dead. Johnny just wouldn't give up. The next day the coach found out about the fight and threw Dennis off the team, saying a senior should know better than to get into a fight with a freshman. I said he should have known better than to get into a fight with a crazy person like Johnny.

As for me, well, I didn't like to fight, however I never backed down if confronted. In the South End of Albany sometimes you had to fight to survive. Somehow, I had this reputation that you didn't mess with Sonny. Maybe it was because some of my family worked for the mob, my Uncle Mickey King ran a gambling operation in the back of his candy store. Maybe it was my size and maybe it was because I had never lost a fight but at any rate, I was respected on the streets.

When we were still in high school, there was an incident one Saturday night at the Arbor Hills Bowling Lanes. Johnny was being loud as usual and somehow he made the mistake of irritating David Greene. David was the meanest and toughest kid in Albany. His mother was Italian and his father was a Jew who owned a local pawn shop. David was 5'11" and about 200lbs with slicked back black hair and a square jaw. He was known and feared by everyone in the South End and Johnny had really ticked him off. Johnny had just picked up his bowling ball and was getting ready to bowl when David came over and asked Johnny to repeat whatever it was he said. Even Johnny knew this was one person he didn't want to fight. It looked like David was serious and unfortunately Tommy wasn't with us to help. I quickly ran over and stood between David and Johnny. It was almost a reflex.

David said, "Sonny, I don't have a beef with you but you better get out of my way. Your little friend just opened his big mouth for the last time."

I don't know what came over me but this shaft of steel firmed up in my backbone and I replied, "David, I don't want to fight you but you'll have to go through me to get to him, now back off!"

To my great relief David said, "Johnny, this is your lucky day. If I didn't like your friend Sonny, you'd be dead. Watch yourself, the next time you won't be so lucky." Then walking away, he turned and said to me, "Sonny, what are you doing hanging out with a loser like Johnny?"

"He's not a loser, he's my friend." I replied. As word of this incident spread, my reputation grew. Thereafter, I never had to worry about anyone disrespecting me on the streets.

Tommy was a war hero. The day after Pearl Harbor was attacked he enlisted in the Navy. He served on the USS Yorktown and received a medal for valor during the Battle of Midway. The Yorktown was torpedoed by a Japanese submarine and the crew had to abandon ship. Many of his shipmates died and many more were injured. Tommy helped save the lives of several men that day. He received 3rd degree burns on parts of both legs and was returned to Pearl Harbor after the battle to recuperate. Three months later after his rehabilitation, he was reassigned to another aircraft carrier and finished out the war with no further incident.

I was very proud of Tommy and wished that I was able to join him. We threw him a great home coming party when he was discharged. Soon after that we went into the scrap business together.

Johnny on the other hand enlisted in the Marines, no surprise there. However, he didn't have the temperament and had a real issue with authority figures. Johnny's old man would beat him on a weekly basis whether he deserved it or not. When he was 16, he'd had enough and fought back, breaking his father's nose. He was thrown out of the house and dropped out of school. He basically lived on the streets from then on. Because of his trouble with his father, he couldn't stand anyone yelling at him. Somehow he made it through boot camp at Paris Island and was assigned to an infantry platoon. His sergeant was trying to make a man out of Johnny and rode him hard every day. Johnny couldn't take it and one day when his sergeant got up into his face screaming at him for being a subpar Marine, Johnny attacked him. Several members of his platoon pulled him off the sergeant and the MPs came and threw Johnny in the brig. Thirty days later he was released with a warning that anymore problems and he would be dishonorably discharged. Well, Johnny had enough and went AWOL. They caught him 2 months later at a bar in the South End. He spent the rest of the war in federal prison. When he got out no one would hire him with his record except this local bookie, Pat Pasquale. Johnny became his errand boy.

After I got sick, both of my friends did their best to help me out. However, when I accepted the Lord I saw less and less of Johnny. When my disease progressed and I became bedridden, he never came by at all. After 1960, I wondered if I would ever see Johnny again. It broke my heart. We were so close, like brothers. I asked Tommy and my Uncle Peter to check on Johnny and to tell him I wanted to see him and that I hoped he was alright. Johnny's response was always the same. "I feel sorry for Frank, but I can't stand all that Jesus stuff. Jesus, Jesus, Jesus, that's all he wants to talk about. It's like he's a different person. No, tell Frank I send my best and hope he gets better." I never stopped praying for Johnny. I prayed that God would open his heart and draw him to Jesus.

Over the years, people would tell me about Johnny, whatever they heard or that they bumped into him. He continued to work for the bookie and in fact eventually had his own bookmaking operation. By the time he was forty he had married and divorced three times and had four kids that he never saw. People told me that he had a serious drinking problem and was abusive to his own kids and wives. History was repeating itself. He apparently was making a lot of money as a bookie and was a big spender. Even though he never saw his own kids, he had attracted several young guys who were impressed by his fancy Cadillac and free spending ways. From time to time my sons would stop by to visit us. One day my youngest, Ricardo, came by with a very disturbing story.

"Dad, guess who I ran into last week." Ricardo began, "An old friend of yours, Johnny Canavi."

I was very upset. I did not want Ricardo to become involved with Johnny. Although I could no longer raise my voice, I said as loud as I could, "Ricardo, do not believe this man. I want you to promise me that you will not see this man again."

Ricardo was surprised by the intensity of my reaction and quickly said, "OK Dad, don't worry, I won't see him. It was a chance meeting anyway. But if you feel that strongly about him then I promise I won't see him again."

I continued to pray for Johnny everyday and hoped that in the future I would see him again as a better man.

Tommy on the other hand was a faithful friend. He had married a beautiful girl from the neighborhood and had three kids. His scrap metal business had expanded and he was now a broker with his own scrap yard down at the Port of Albany on the Hudson River. People from all over upstate New York would bring scrap to him that he would buy and then sell at a profit. Even with his busy schedule, he still found the time to visit me once or twice every month. Knowing how tight our finances were he always brought bags of groceries and insisted that my mother take them. At first, he tried to give her cash but her reaction was so strong that he respected her wishes and instead brought groceries

Tommy had always been a good Catholic and didn't really understand my "new religion" but he was respectful. As I did with everyone who visited me, I asked him to do me a favor and as was always the case he said that he would. My favor was for him to be my hands and write a letter for me. What could he say? This was my crafty way to witness to the people and also get my ministry letters written.

Tommy would often have questions about what I asked him to write. I would tell him where to look in the Bible to back up some of the points of my letters. We had wonderful discussions about the Lord. It was a blessing for me to share my love of the Lord with my good friend. This went on for several years.

Then one day, Tommy said, "Frank, I've been reading the Bible and I have a question."

I replied, "What is it Tommy? You seem so serious."

"Frank, how do you know if you are saved? I've always had this fear that someday I would die with a mortal sin on my soul and go to hell." He confided.

I told him, "Tommy, God is a God of grace and mercy. He wants us to have blessed assurance and to be secure in our salvation." He nodded his understanding as he looked intently at me.

I continued, "Do you believe in God and in His son Jesus Christ?"

"Yes I do." He replied.

"Do you acknowledge that you are a sinner in need of a Savior who is Jesus and are you sorry for your sins and ask God to forgive you?" I asked.

Tommy said, "Yes I do, Lord please forgive me."

Then I said, "Do you accept Jesus as your Lord and Savior and do you invite Him into your heart?"

Tommy's eyes welled up with tears saying, "Lord Jesus come into my heart."

I told Tommy that he could be assured that he was saved and that no matter what, that the Lord was faithful and his sins were forgiven and nothing and no one could ever separate him from God's love.

Tommy left our apartment that day beaming. The love of God was all over him. I felt so blessed that God would use me to lead my friend to Him.

Three days later the doorbell rang in the afternoon. My mother was preparing dinner and we were not expecting any visitors. I heard an unfamiliar voice talking to my mother in the kitchen. This man whom I hadn't seen in 10 years followed my mother into the room. At first I did not recognize him. It was David Greene. The years had not been kind to him. Yes, he still looked like someone who you would not want to mess with but he looked much older than his years.

"Frank, how are you doing? I've wanted to come by here many times but I just didn't know what to say." He said.

"David, I'm surprised by your visit. We knew each other but we weren't exactly friends. Not that I'm not glad to see you." His visit indeed was a surprise. Over the years from time to time someone would mention David and it always involved something very bad. Tommy once told me that his wife saw David beating up this man on South Pearl Street. Apparently, the man owed money to David's boss and either wouldn't or couldn't pay up. Tommy's wife started to yell at David to leave this guy alone and when he wouldn't, she went and found a cop, who finally made him stop. The local cops knew all about David and feared him as did everyone in the South End. David was a leg breaker for the local mob, an enforcer and from what I heard he was very good at his job. The rumor was that he killed several men and not only worked for the mob but he was also on loan to the local political machine for strong arm work. Because of all these stories I was led by the Holy Spirit to pray for David and had done so on a regular basis for years. Even so, I was very surprised to see David Greene moving a chair to sit close to my bed.

"Frank, I'm sure you'll hear this soon and I don't know why I feel so compelled to be the one to tell you but I have some bad news." He paused and looked down at the floor. I was busting by this time. What in the world could he be getting at? He looked up and said, "Frank, its Tommy Phelan, I was over near his business earlier today. Apparently, he was working in his scrap yard. There were a couple of tons of scrap piled against a wall. Tommy was next to the pile looking for something with his back to the wall and somehow the pile of scrap collapsed on top of him. He's dead. Frank, I know how close you two were. I'm sorry and if there is something I can do, please let me know."

Tears began to well up in my eyes and the Lord quickly reminded me that three days earlier Tommy had accepted the Lord. Tommy had gone home and was now in Paradise with the Lord.

I responded, "David, thank you for your concern and kindness but Tommy is in a better place and I'm confident that the Lord will take care of his family. It will all be alright."

David seemed surprised by my answer and said, "Frank, would you mind if I stopped by for a visit once in a while?" Sensing that the Lord was at work, I encouraged him to do so.

Losing Tommy was very hard for me. The McGraw brothers carried me to the funeral. Tommy's wife and children were inconsolable. It all happened so suddenly. She came from a large close knit family and would receive all the support she needed. Now he was gone. I missed him so very much. Tommy had been a great friend but I was comforted by the fact that one day I would see him again in heaven.

A few weeks later David Greene returned. We talked about how life sure wasn't turning out like we expected. He asked me, "Frank, how do you do it? How do you lay there on your bed, hour after hour, day by day? That would drive me crazy."

I explained, "David, I'm able to do it only with the help of Jesus. Without him I'd be lost and with him all thing are possible."

"I'd heard that you became very religious. I don't think that's for me. I'm afraid I'm beyond help. I haven't been to church or synagogue in twenty years." He said.

"David, no one is beyond hope or too far gone for the Lord to help. I don't care what you've done and by the way I don't consider myself religious. I'm not religious, that has to do with a lot of rules and regulations, but I am in a relationship with Jesus Christ my Lord. This may surprise you but I've been praying for you for over 10 years now." I told him.

"Oh really, and what have you been praying for?" David asked with a bit of sarcasm.

I replied, "Well, I've heard some pretty bad things about you over the years. I'm not saying I believe all these rumors but just in case, I've been praying that you would repent and change your life."

"Frank, I've probably done worse things than what you've heard. I've killed people. Does that shock you? I'm a lost cause." He stated.

I explained to him about another murderer I knew. His name was David too and he was the apple of God's eye. And then I told him about yet another murderer named Moses. God used him to deliver a nation out of bondage. I concluded saying, "David, no one is beyond God's mercy and grace."

When David left that day, I felt that the Lord was working on him, drawing him to Jesus. I continued to pray for him. A week later he returned. He sat down next to the bed and said, "Frank, I want what you have. I can't go on living with all the stuff that I've done. I need to have that relationship with Jesus, if he will accept me. What do I have to do to be saved?"

"Praise God!" I said. "Hold my hand and let's pray, repeat after me. Lord Jesus, I am a sinner. I am sorry for all my sins. Please forgive me, come into my heart and Lord Jesus…."

David had been repeating this sinners' prayer and at this point he jumped to his feet and shouted at the top of his lungs, "LORD JESUS!!!

LORD JESUS!!!" The Holy Spirit had convicted him and David had received the Baptism of Spirit right then and there. My mother and father, on hearing this commotion, came running into the room. My mother had seen this before and she started praising God as was I. The Spirit was so strong in the room that it felt as if the building was shaking. My mother called Brother Anthony and asked him to come over immediately. The Lord's move was so powerful that she felt we needed a Christian of Brother Anthony's maturity to help David.

David was on fire for the Lord. When Brother Anthony arrived, he prayed for wisdom and prayed that the Lord would protect David from the enemy. David had been an agent of Satan and the devil would not take kindly when one of his own switched sides to play for the Lord.

Over the next several weeks David indeed was a new creation. He went to all his old haunts; the bars, brothels etc. and began to witness, calling for his one-time partners in sin to repent and accept Jesus. David tried to witness to a bouncer at a nightclub he used to frequent. This man had a score to settle with David. His new love for the Lord was seen as weakness by the bouncer. He beat David so badly that he was in the hospital for a week. David refused to fight back. As soon as he was released from the hospital, he went back to that nightclub and told the bouncer that not only did he forgive him but that Jesus would too. The bouncer spit in his face and kicked him out of the club.

Sometime later, David, who was now a member of the New Albany Church of God, came to see me. He told me that the Holy Spirit was prompting him to go to the police department and confess his crimes. He said that although he probably wouldn't see me again in this life that he would always think about me and pray for me.

David was obedient to the Lord's leading and confessed to all his crimes. Because of his confession, the judge had mercy on him and sentenced him to life without parole sending him to Sing Sing State Prison in Ossining, New York. I heard that soon after entering the prison, David began a prison ministry and was preaching to the other inmates. I recalled that incident in the bowling alley so many years ago. I never knew why David backed down when I stepped between him and Johnny Canavi. Now I understood that even back then God was weaving his miracle, Praise God!

CHAPTER 10

THE TRACH

Looking back on it, I guess I should have expected this would happen. Dr. Macumber told me that it would be a possibility. Even so, I still was not prepared. Wasn't it enough that I couldn't move my arms and legs, my hands and feet? I could barely turn my head to look out the window. If a fly landed on my nose, I wasn't able to swat it away. Wasn't that enough helplessness? And now I was congested. I no longer had the ability to cough. I couldn't blow my nose. The mucus was building up in my lungs and it was choking me. Dr. Macumber said the MS could progress to the point that my throat muscles could become paralyzed.

My mother had not slept through the night since I had to move back home ten years ago. She always got up at 12, 2 and 4am to be sure I was doing OK. It was just past three when I woke up unable to breathe. My cold was worse and the mucus was so thick that it was blocking my windpipe. My mother had not gone back to sleep since checking on me at 2am. She heard me wheeze and rushed into my room.

We had Dr. Macumber's home phone number. He was so concerned about me and was always available to help. My mother called him and blurted out in a frantic voice, "Doctor, this is Mary, Frank can't breathe. He's all congested and I don't know what to do! Help us, please help us!" By this time my father was up and in the room.

"Mary, listen to me, try to calm down, he's going to be alright." Dr. Macumber assured.

My mother interrupted and started to scream, "He can't breathe! He stopped breathing!"

"Mary, is Frank wheezing? Are there any gasping sounds?" The doctor asked.

She replied, "No, no, he can't breathe!"

Dr. Macumber had two lines on his phone for such emergencies and had his wife call the hospital while he stayed on the phone with my mother.

"Mary, listen to me carefully. An ambulance is on the way but you don't have time to wait. Get a small sharp knife, the sharpest you have." He told her. My mother was frantic and shouted to my father to get the knife.

"You have straws for Frank to drink, get two of them now." The doctor instructed. My mother kept straws on a table near my bed. The only way I could drink liquids was through a straw. She tried to remain calm and told the doctor she had the knife and straws in hand.

Dr. Macumber instructed her to remove any pillows behind my head so that she could tilt my head back. "Now find the indentation just below Frank's Adam's apple. Have you found it?"

"Yes, I've got it." She replied.

"Now, make a half-inch incision across, not up or down, and go a half-inch deep. He'll bleed but don't worry, it shouldn't bleed too much." He told her.

My mother handed the phone to my father and prepared to cut me. She hesitated but knew that if she didn't do this, then I would die by drowning in my own mucus. She asked Jesus for help to steady her hand and then she took the knife and attempted to make the incision. Nothing happened, she didn't go deep enough. My father was telling the doctor what was happening and told him that it didn't work. Dr. Macumber said for her to try again but she had to stick the knife in my throat a half an inch. She took a deep breath, said another prayer and stuck the knife the required depth and cut across a half an inch. Blood began to run down my neck onto the sheets. At the sight of my blood, my mother began to panic. The doctor assured my father that this was OK and not to worry. My father acting as the go between told my mother what Dr. Macumber was saying.

"Pinch the incision open and put both straws into the incision about one inch deep. Breathe into the straws with two quick breaths. Now wait five seconds and do one breath into the straws every five seconds." My father related, repeating Dr. Macumber's orders.

My mother followed his instructions and I started to regain consciousness. My chest began to rise and fall. It wasn't easy but I was able to breathe on my own. My mother was so relieved that she began to sob and praise Jesus. I was unable to speak but in my mind, I too was praising the Lord. Just about then the door bell rang and the ambulance arrived.

The ambulance driver and an emergency technician were prepared to replace the straws with a temporary trach and air tubes. They cleaned me up and moved me onto a stretcher to take me to the hospital. The driver asked my mother if she did the incision. She replied that she did. He complimented her on the job she did and told her that she saved my life. She said, "No, it wasn't me, the Lord Jesus saved him."

As the emergency technicians carried me downstairs to the ambulance, I lost consciousness again. The ordeal had been too much. In my unconscious state the Lord allowed me full use and control of my body, at least in my mind. I dreamt I was in Lincoln Park with my three boys. I was young again and the boys were still little. We were playing tag and I was it. As I chased my sons they were laughing uncontrollably. When I caught up with one of the boys we would fall to the ground and I would tickle them. The other two boys would then jump on top of me. They laughed until they cried. It was pure joy. There was no thought of sickness. The Lord would often bless me with these beautiful thoughts. Unfortunately, I would then wake up.

I was in the hospital for a week as they repaired the emergency incision that my mother made. A permanent trach was put in place. She saved my life and I was grateful but it was a messy job. The knife and the straws that she used were not sterile and the area around the incision as well as my wind pipe became infected. This would become a constant problem with the trach. Despite my mother's best efforts to keep everything sterile, that area around the trach would continually become infected. When I couldn't cough up mucus, which was several times every day, the mucus would block my windpipe. My mother and sometimes my father would use a suction tube attached to a machine to clear my throat. They would check on this many times every day. Later, when I was moved to the convalescent home, the staff was not as diligent. This made my life even more difficult.

Up until this time, even though I was now completely paralyzed, occasionally I was able to get out of the house. I especially enjoyed going to church on Sunday and seeing my brothers and sisters at the New Albany Church of God. I always enjoyed hearing Brother Anthony's sermons. They really lifted my spirit. He would try to drop by every week to encourage me, and that was a blessing, but it was not the same as getting out and going to church. The trach, the tubes and the suction machine made it too difficult to go anyplace, not to mention that I was now much more vulnerable to catching colds, viruses and the flu. Anything like that could be fatal to me. I would have pneumonia at least a dozen times in the following years. When I got pneumonia, Dr. Macumber always insisted that I go to the hospital. Several times I almost died but the Lord was not ready for me to come home. My witness here on earth still wasn't finished. I felt like Paul, who wrote in Philippians, "For to me, to live is Christ and to die is gain. If I am to go on living in the body, this will mean fruitful labor for me. Yet what shall I choose? I do not know! I am torn between the two: I desire to depart and be with Christ, which is better by far; but it is more necessary for you that I remain in the body. Convinced of this, I know that I will remain, and I will continue with all of you for your progress and joy in the faith, so that through my being with you again your joy in Christ Jesus will overflow on account of me." Now, I am not comparing myself to Paul, but I can understand his feelings and like Paul, for now I know that I will remain for the glory of Jesus Christ.

CHAPTER 11

MY THREE SONS

The Apostle Paul wrote to the Philippians, "But one thing I do: Forgetting what is behind and straining toward what is ahead, I press on toward the goal to win the prize for which God has called me heavenward in Jesus Christ."

I was able to live according to Paul's advice and example for the most part. But sometimes I couldn't help but have regrets about my kids. I missed not being there for them. My two sons from my first marriage, Bobby and Frank Jr. had to grow up in an orphanage, LaSalle School for Boys. I heard that the Christian Brothers at LaSalle were kind but very strict.

Ricardo's mother, Rosie, eventually remarried and I didn't really know how that was for him. Was the stepfather a good man? Was he a good father? I never really knew. When I asked Ricardo how things were at home, he would always reply, "Everything is fine." I was grateful knowing that Ricardo was being provided for. Sometimes I gave in to envy, thinking that another man had taken my place. I tried not to dwell on such things that were beyond my control. All I could do was to give it over to the Lord and trust that He would take care of all things.

My mother and father never really encouraged the boys to come over the house to visit me. They had their hands full, so I can't really fault them. Taking care of me was a full time job for my mother. That left it up to my father to earn enough money to support the three of us. A tailor working in a small men's clothing store did not make a lot of money. We did receive a small disability check each month from the government. This helped but with all my medical expenses it was very difficult. The sicker I got, the less I saw of my boys.

Bobby and Frankie's grandmother on their mother's side was very kind, unlike her daughter who hadn't seen the boys in years and didn't care to. Their grandmother, Mrs. Murphy, would drive the boys to our house every few months and leave them for a several hours before picking them up and returning to LaSalle. However, my mother was not as loving as she might have been to the older two boys. She would make comments about how she suspected that Frankie in particular was not my son. She remembered the lost little boy who was always getting into trouble and not the man that he might become. I knew he was my son. He looked just like me but my mother for all her devotion to me, just never accepted him. After Frankie graduated from high school he came by the house. He had been working down at the Port of Albany loading and unloading trucks. He wasn't making a lot of money but he tried to give my mother some of the little he had. My mother refused and flew off the handle. She asked him where he got this money, implying that he stole the money. Her reasoning was that this young man, who once stole money from his teacher's pocketbook when he was 5 years old, couldn't possibly earn an honest dollar. I saw the dejected look on his face. I didn't have the strength in my vocal cords to protest and defend my son. This young man who had been rejected all his life was trying to help us out and in doing so, perhaps gain acceptance from a family that never really wanted him. I recalled the terrible scene in my kitchen when I first got sick. That dark day my parents took the boys to go live at LaSalle. Oh how Frankie screamed and fought to stay with us, how he pleaded and begged but to no avail. He desperately wanted to be part of a family and once again that family said no.

I remember the last time I saw my son Frankie. It was shortly after my mother refused to take any money from him. It was an afternoon in the middle of the week, it was in the fall. Apparently Frankie had very little contact with my youngest son Ricardo. They hadn't seen each other in years. Ricardo's stepfather apparently didn't encourage him to bring friends into his house and for sure didn't want Ricardo's half brother around. Because of the infrequent visits to our apartment by the boys, their paths hadn't crossed in many years. When Ricardo was about 11 years old, he received a letter from Frankie. In the letter Frankie began, "Ricky, please read this letter real good and then give it to your mother to read." In the letter, Frankie was again pleading for someone to love him. He begged Ricardo to intercede with Rosie to let him come live with them. If Rosie couldn't handle being his mother when he was 6 years old, she sure wouldn't do it when he was 13 years old. I found out about this after Ricardo told my mother about this letter. When Ricardo's stepfather found the letter he tore it up and threw it away.

Now Frankie was 18 and Ricardo was 16 and hadn't seen or spoken to each other for several years. Somehow Frankie found out that Ricardo was playing football for his high school and was practicing at the fields in Lincoln Park, the same fields that I used to bring the three boys to play when I could still walk. Ricardo noticed this older boy standing on the sidelines watching practice and that he seemed a little out of place because he was all dressed up in a fancy suit.

After practice Frankie went up to Ricardo as he was walking off the field and identified himself as his brother. Ricardo later told us that he didn't know what to do. He knew he could not bring him back to his house as his stepfather wouldn't tolerate that. We lived in an apartment on the other side of Lincoln Park, a couple of miles from where Ricardo lived with his mother and step father. Ricardo suggested that he and Frankie come to our apartment. I remember the day well because it was so awkward. I was not able to speak very well and Ricardo just wanted to leave and go home without Frankie. Frankie suggested that he would like to go home with Ricardo and maybe he could spend the night. Ricardo knew that if he brought Frankie home, it would mean trouble.

Now that Frankie was out of school and was 18 years old, he could no longer stay at LaSalle. He had been living wherever someone would let him sleep on a couch or sometimes at the YMCA on a cot. Apparently, this had been going on for several months and he was really desperate. Finally, Ricardo made up some excuse and left our apartment. Ten minutes later, so did Frankie, rejected again.

I heard that a week or so later Frankie enlisted in the army. Apparently, his Uncle Sam had a place for him. I never saw him again. Several years passed by and we found out that Frankie was living in the San Francisco area and working for Bobby in the restaurant business. His brother Bobby was always there for him and perhaps the only family he ever really knew. Whether he found the acceptance he so desperately craved with a wife and children of his own, I can only pray that he did. Yes, regarding Frankie I always had regrets.

My oldest son Bobby somehow handled his childhood or lack of childhood somewhat better than Frankie. If he experienced the same inner turmoil of having no permanent family presence, he didn't let it show. He became a basketball star for LaSalle averaging over 20 points per game. Upon graduation, he enlisted in the Air Force. Even my mother couldn't help but be proud when Bobby came by to visit wearing his beautiful dress uniform. Bobby was assigned to Air Force Intelligence. A man who worked for the State Dept. came by the apartment to ask several questions about Bobby's background. Apparently, Bobby's new position required a higher level of security clearance. While stationed in Puerto Rico, Bobby met a beautiful Puerto Rican girl. They got married and within three years they had two children, a boy and a girl. I never met Bobby's wife or my grandchildren but at least he sent photos of his family. Bobby was stationed out of the country most of the time and I guess it was difficult for him to come back to Albany. Eventually, he left the service and made his way to California with his family. I never found out why he went out there. I think he resolved in his mind that he really didn't have family here. He had relations but not family and unlike Frankie, he determined that he didn't need us. You can't really blame him. We never exactly showered him with love. I eased my conscience about the childhood my children endured by telling myself that if only I had not gotten sick, things would have been different. If only.....

I probably saw my youngest son Ricardo more than the other two boys over the years. As expected however, the older he grew, the less I saw of him. When he was 6 years old, we moved to a cheaper apartment close to Lincoln Park. He lived with his mother and her family and eventually his stepfather in an apartment on the other side of the park, maybe 3 miles away. He would come over to visit one Sunday each month even though no one from his mother's side of his family would drive him. This little boy would walk through the park the whole way. When it was time for him to go home, my mother would call a cab and give Ricky two dollars, a lot of money to her, to take the cab home. He would never complain about anything. When I asked him how things were at home, he would always reply that they were fine. He loved the San Francisco Giants and one of my few pleasures in life besides the Lord of course, was discussing the Giants and their chances to win the Pennant. He especially idolized Willie Mays. Ricardo's childhood was far more stable than Bobby and Frankie, yet I sensed a real sadness in his heart. I witnessed to him about the Lord many times as I did the other boys and he would always be polite. I remember giving him a Bible for Christmas. My mother had his name engraved on the black Bible cover in gold lettering. He seemed disappointed that this was his Christmas present. However, we are to plant seeds and rely on the Holy Spirit to stimulate growth in His good time. Ricardo grew to be an excellent athlete in high school and played on the varsity basketball and football teams. He was a fine looking young man. He went to college in Alabama where he met his future wife. After school he and his wife moved to Albany for a time in the early 70's. This was just before I was moved to the convalescent home. I was very disappointed that he never brought his wife by to meet me. It really hurt me. The only time I saw him during this period was when I was in the hospital for one of my many bouts with pneumonia. On that occasion, they really thought I was going to die and indeed I almost did but the Lord still had work for me to do. One of the ladies from the church went to Albany Savings Bank where Ricky was working and told him that he really needed to come to the hospital after work as I didn't have much longer to live. He did come to the hospital to see me but only stayed for a brief visit. I'm afraid he came more out of obligation than real concern. I surprised everyone and survived and when my fever broke and I was coming around, my mother told me I was praising Jesus.

I didn't see Ricardo again for three years. He had moved to Alabama but he did return to Albany to visit his mother and her family. By then I was living in the Albany County home. Rosie's brother Pat had become a strong Spirit filled Christian. He would visit me from time to time. Pat came to see me and to my delight brought Ricardo and his little son, my grandson, Zachary. We had a very nice visit for about an hour. I couldn't help to think how wonderful it might have been if only I had not gotten sick. If only I was healthy, then I would be taking my grandson to see a baseball game or to the zoo instead of watching him fidget and asking his father, "Can we go now?" I understood of course, after all he was only 3 years old, but it was one more hurt, one more disappointment.

I never saw or heard from Ricardo again. They had moved back to Alabama, far enough away to not have to care about me. If only I had not gotten sick. Lord, why did this have to happen?

There wasn't a single day that I didn't lift my sons up in prayer. I prayed that the Lord would draw them to Jesus and that they would spend their lives following him. I prayed that they would be strong in the Lord and that their lives would be a blessing to others and glorify God. I prayed for God's tender mercy in allowing me to see the answer to that prayer.

CHAPTER 12

HOW LONG, O LORD, HOW LONG

In Psalm 6, David writes,

> "Be merciful to me, Lord, for I am faint;
> O Lord, heal me, for my bones are in agony.
> My soul is in anguish.
> How long, O Lord, how long?
>
> Turn, O Lord, and deliver me;
> save me because of your unfailing love.
>
> I am worn out from groaning;
> All night long I flood my bed with weeping
> And drench my couch with tears.
> My eyes grow weak with sorrow"

Daily, I read the Book of Psalms, imploring the Lord for relief but to no avail. The only answer I received from the Holy Spirit was, "My grace is sufficient." By 1975 times became very difficult for us. My mother was growing older. For 20 years she faithfully cared for me, day and night she cared for me. The strain, however, was getting to be too much for her. From time to time she would get sick herself. She had high blood pressure and her heart was weak. During these times when she was unable to take care of me, my father and Aunt Camille would fill in.

One afternoon, my mother was resting on a chair in my room. My trach needed to be suctioned so she called my father to help out. The stress of having a sick wife and son and still having to go to the tailor shop everyday at 75 years of age was too much. He came into my room and shouted, "Mary, I can't take this anymore. It would be better for everyone if he would just go ahead and die!"

My mother did not need this anxiety on top of all her other problems. She started to sob and replied to him, "No, No, No!" She cried. "How dare you say that, don't ever say that again! Frank, don't listen to him!"

My father suctioned my trach and just walked out of the room without saying another word. We all were at the breaking point. During the past few months, I overheard friends and family talking to my mother in the kitchen. I could still hear pretty well. They would suggest that maybe it was time for me to go live in the county home. It was very difficult for me to speak. I could whisper my words and sometimes there would be no sound at all and I would only mouth my words. My mother had gotten quite good at understanding me. It was almost as if she could read my mind. She bent over my bed and gave me her full attention and I said, "Ma, you have got to put me in the home."

Years earlier, when I was still in a wheelchair, I had gone to the Albany County Convalescent Home to minister to the residents. I remembered how bad that place was and dreaded the thought of going there but as bad as that prospect was, I could no longer bear to watch my mother slowly die from the stress of caring for me.

She refused to listen to me. "Frank, now don't you start. What would I do without you?" She replied. My mother had given me her constant attention for over 20 years. The visiting nurses and Dr Macumber were amazed at the condition of my skin. I never had bed sores because my mother would move me from side to side and to my back several times every day, sometimes every hour. I was no longer a big man but this was still a lot of weight for an old woman to handle. She would keep large pillows situated between my legs so that my knees and ankles would not rub together. This helped reduce the possibility of sores. She had this electric messaging device that fit on her hand. Every day she would message my head, neck, back, arms and legs to keep the blood circulation going. She would make me eat the good food that she lovingly prepared and made me drink plenty of water as this also helped to reduce bed sores. After she bathed and shaved me, she would moisturize my skin with lotion. As a result, except for my frequent bouts with pneumonia, I was doing as well as possible, under the circumstances.

One morning all that changed. My mother always came into my room at 6 AM. That day was different. By 7 she still hadn't come in. Suddenly, I heard my father screaming, "Mary, Mary, wake up!" I knew something was very wrong and immediately begged God to help her. Soon after that I heard a siren as an ambulance arrived.

I could hear the emergency technicians trying to revive my mother. They hurried her out of the apartment and within minutes the siren was blaring again and they were on their way to the hospital. My Aunt Camille came in and told me that my mother had a heart attack but that she was still breathing. She held my hand and we prayed. Camille was a very powerful Christian woman, full of the Holy Spirit. Having her there with me was the only way I think I could have gotten through this. I was worried sick and couldn't eat at all that day. Camille told me that she and my mother had talked about this possibility and that she promised her that she would stay with me, at least until some situation could be arranged for me. Unfortunately, I knew what that arrangement would be.

My father spent the nights at the hospital and would come by my room and tell me about my mother. "Frank, they performed open heart surgery and the doctors are hopeful she will live," he began. "But Frank, I must prepare you for some bad news. Your mother must rest. She will not be able to care for you as she has in the past. Your Aunt Camille has her own problems and I have to work, our finances are drained and I cannot retire. Forgive me son but I have talked to Social Services and they are going to move you to the county home. Maybe it will only be temporary. I just don't know what else to do."

I could see tears welling up in his eyes. Although my mother bore the brunt of my care, his life had been hard and bitter as well. A man in his mid 70's should not have to work as hard as he does. He patted my head and left the room. Camille was waiting in the kitchen while my father broke the news to me. She had been crying and told me that God would not forget me. "Frank, Jesus will never leave you or forsake you. You believe that don't you." I mouthed "yes" that I did and I said, "Praise God."

The next morning an ambulance came to the house and two men in white jackets lifted me onto a stretcher and carried me out of the apartment to transport me to the county home. Other than living with MS, my greatest fear was now being realized. "Lord Jesus, I need you even more. You've told me that your grace is sufficient for me. Please give me abundant grace now." My father had to be at work but Camille followed the ambulance in her car.

When we arrived at the county home, I was brought into a small hospital room. "You're lucky Mr. Angelo," said one of the ambulance workers, "you have a private room. There aren't many single bed units in this place." I thought to myself, yeah, I'm really lucky.

The first thing I noticed was how cold the room was. I was given a sheet and a thin blanket and that was it. When I had been here years before, it was in the spring time and much more comfortable. Maybe I'll get used to it. I could see that the walls hadn't been painted in many years and the faded gray paint was peeling in several places. The musty smell of the room was thick and testified to the overall cleanliness or lack of cleanliness of the room. My Aunt Camille just shook her head and said, "Frank, I'm so sorry about this. I just don't know what else to do. It's a bit chilly in here, I'll bring some blankets by tomorrow.

After Camille left, I laid there on my back for what seemed like several hours before a nurse's aide came into the room. She was in a big hurry as she helped me drink some water and spooned what tasted like baby food into my mouth. She hardly spoke and spent only about 10 minutes in my room and then was gone. She didn't turn me and left me lying there on my back. The next day my father came by and I tried to explain that the nurses only came by a few times and turned me just once. He said that the county home did not receive enough money to operate the facility. As a result, they were understaffed and the people who worked here were underpaid. He said that Camille had already complained to the administrator but his response was that they were doing the very best they could with the resources they had and he would try to have someone check in on me as much as possible.

My father tried to come by every other day or so. The news about my mother was good and bad. The good news was she had survived the heart attack. The bad news, the doctor insisted that she get as much rest as possible with absolutely no exertion. The doctor told my father that her next heart attack would kill her for sure. After she was released from the hospital, my mother came to see me. Brother Anthony came with her. She was now confined to her own wheelchair and Brother Anthony wheeled her into my room. Within seconds, she began to sob after seeing me and the conditions I was now living in. My blanket had slipped off me and she could see the bed sores. She could see and smell the unclean room and could feel the lack of heat. "Frank, I'm so sorry." She sobbed.

Seeing me like this was just too difficult for her. She still managed to come at least once a week. She would always bring someone who was strong enough to turn me.

Over the next few months, I came to realize just how good I had it when I was living at home, when my mother was able to take such good care of me. Besides the bedsores, my catheter was always left in me too long and not cleaned properly. Twice my drainage bag was not changed in time and my urine backed up into my bladder causing a nasty urinary tract and blood infection. On top of that, a few of the nurses and aides were verbally abusive and were very rough when they had to clean me. Bathing me was very inconvenient for them and was never done well. As a result I stunk and just the thought of that made me very uncomfortable. Suctioning my trach was only done when someone would come into my room those few times every day. Breathing was very difficult and was something that I struggled with each day.

I remembered what my father said to my mother before her heart attack, "It would be better for everyone if he would just go ahead and die." "Lord, I'm ready to go, please take me." I prayed.

PART II

WHAT COULD HAVE BEEN

CHAPTER 13

THE SECOND CHANCE

"It would be better for everyone if he would just go ahead and die." My father's words replayed over and over in my mind as I woke up in my room at the county home. I must have been unconscious for awhile. I was no longer lying in my own filth. Apparently someone had come in and cleaned me up. Reliving the past twenty plus years had drained me. For whatever reason, I was just given a view of my years of suffering. I was overwhelmed with the feeling that my life had been denied to me and was wasted. On top of that, the lives of those I loved were damaged irreparably. My mother exhausted her life caring for me. She hadn't slept more than two consecutive hours in 20 years. My father was a poor old bitter man. Any plans he had of prosperity, of owning his own tailor shop, disappeared with my illness. My two oldest sons were raised in an orphanage. My youngest boy was raised by another man who may or may not have cared for him.

The blessings, my relationship with the Lord, all the people I may have helped to know Jesus, His grace that really had been sufficient for me, was forgotten. What about me, why did I have to suffer this way. Couldn't I have helped more people if I had not been sick? A feeling swept over me that I had not experienced since receiving that terrible diagnosis all those years ago that I had MS. It was a feeling of resentment. Everything was bearable when I was still living at home but now this was more than I could bear.

Not having the physical capacity to shout at God, I began to cry out in my mind. "Why God, why did you make me go through this? In the Bible you healed everyone who called out to you. Why wouldn't you heal me? Look at my family! Look at my sons! Why should they suffer? Why did you let all this happen to me?"

Suddenly, my eyesight grew dim, more than faded, I was blind. It happened so fast, it was as if someone had turned the lights off in a darkened cellar without windows. My sight had been fading in and out for 20 years. It was part of the MS but not like this. I thought to myself that now I was going to be punished for being angry with God. I said, "God, please don't take my sight as well."

Just as suddenly, I was surrounded by brilliant light, more brilliant than the sunniest summer day at the beach. My entire being was seized with fear as this indescribable presence stood before me. I tried to speak but could not. The presence began to speak, not audibly but to my mind.

"Frank, my son, I have come to you in response to your cries. For twenty years you have suffered and I have told you that my grace was sufficient for you. You have always accepted that answer... until now," said the Lord.

"Lord," I replied. "Surely, you can understand my despair, my discouragement?"

"My son, you have endured much and have been faithful. Because of your faithfulness, I am going to give you the gift of knowledge. The knowledge of what your life would have been had you not gotten sick. You will live your life over as a healthy man. I will send you back to the day you went to the doctor and received that terrible diagnosis. This time however, you will be handed a reprieve, not a death sentence. All knowledge of the life you have lived, all remembrance of your sufferings, will be wiped out and with that, all the wisdom you have gained through your suffering." Having received this word, I passed into oblivion as an image of an hourglass being turned over burned into my mind.

Rosie and I were led to Dr. Macumber's back office. He stood as we entered and asked us to take a seat as he sat down on his plush leather chair behind his large mahogany desk. Leaning forward and looking very somber he began, "Sonny, Rosie, as you know we ran just about every test available that would address your symptoms and everything came back normal. Dr. Paduka and I were quite concerned. With your symptoms, we were afraid of some neurological disease such as Multiple Sclerosis but thank God, all the tests ruled that out."

A wave of relief came flooding over us. "Doctor, this numbness and fatigue. What do you think is wrong?" I asked.

"Sonny, the human body is a complex biological entity. Sometimes we just can't pinpoint the cause. The numbness could be from some superficial nerve damage. You might have injured yourself lifting all that scrap metal with Tommy. I just don't know. But I'll bet that within a week or so you'll be just fine." Dr. Macumber explained.

As we walked out of the doctor's office, Rosie and I hugged. A great weight had been lifted from us. These last 10 days, waiting for the results of the tests had been hell, but now I felt like a man on death row who just received a pardon. The doctor was right, by the next week I felt fine. I was able to work just as hard as before I began feeling sick and tired. I know Tommy was relieved to have his partner back up and running. The numbness was gone and my strength had returned.

That day after we came home from the doctor's office, I took Rosie and the boys to Lincoln Park. I felt so energized and relieved by the doctor's good news. What a time we had. We played tag and I would chase the boys and then they would chase me. I would let them catch me and when they did, I fell to the ground and they would all jump on top of me. They laughed so hard they were almost crying. How young and free we felt.

Life was good. The scrap metal business was doing well and was about to do a lot better. We received a call from Abe Sokol, our main scrap dealer down at the docks at the Port of Albany. He told us that the old Freihofer Bakery Building on Spruce Street was about to go up for sale. Freihofer's was relocating to a newer state of the art building in Troy. Most of the ovens and machinery were antiquated and would be left in the old bakery. The owners of Freihofer's wanted the building cleaned out. They thought it might make it easier to sell the place. If Tommy and I wanted the job, Abe could get us the contract to salvage all the scrap. Then we would deliver it to Abe and he would sell the scrap.

Freihofer wanted the building cleared in 30 days. For a job this big we needed help. We hired a few friends as helpers including Johnny Canavi. We worked 12 to 14 hour days every day that month, except for two Sundays and stripped the bakery clean. Abe warned us, that for this job we couldn't cheat. This advice from the man that we always paid extra to look the other way. When we found an old water heater we would fill it up with cement. Now, normally a water heater weighed about 100 lbs but filled with cement they weighed 500 lbs. We were paid by the pound for scrap iron so when our truck was weighed, that cement really increased our total. We didn't consider it cheating so much as getting our fair share. I mean, they were cheating us by paying so little for the scrap, so this made everything even.

We paid our three helpers $200 per week and still Tommy and I cleared $10,000 that month. Adding that to what we had been able to save the past year, we were doing well, quite well indeed. 1953 was a very good year.

CHAPTER 14

THE BAKERY LOUNGE

"Fear God and keep his commandments,
For this is the whole duty of man.
For God will bring every deed into judgment,
Including every hidden thing,
Whether it is good or evil. (Eccles 12: 13–14)

If someone asked me what my dream job would be, other than being a professional singer, my answer would be to own and manage a nightclub. This would give me the opportunity to sing whenever I wanted to. With the money we made pulling the scrap out of the Freihofer building, our dream was about to become a reality.

As we were finishing our work on the Freihofer job, Tommy said, "You know, Sonny, this building would make a great club or restaurant. Look at all this space in here and there is plenty of parking. We always talked about opening our own place some day."

"You're right," I replied and said, "I overheard Abe Sokol mention that the owners of Freihofer were very anxious to sell this place. Let's contact them and see just how much they want for the building. We can go to Mr. Birch at State Bank and see if he'll lend us some money for equipment and give us a mortgage for the building. He helped us when we bought the truck. I'm sure we have enough money for a good down payment. We can do this."

The location was perfect. The neighborhood was a mix of commercial buildings, a couple of businesses and a few blocks away there was a nice residential area. It was exactly the type of building and area we needed. If we had to open a place down around Beaver and State Street or "The Gut" as it was known, we may as well open a dive. The area around the old Freihofer building wasn't populated by prostitutes, gamblers and other hustlers like "The Gut". We envisioned a classy place and such a place would fit nicely into this building and neighborhood. It was just the kind of operation that Mr. Birch might finance for us.

Jack Freihofer was the new president of the company. He was the grandson of the company founder. We got his phone number from Abe Sokol and called him about buying the building. He seemed very receptive and asked us to come to his new office in Troy to discuss terms. Tommy and I both wore white shirts and striped business ties, sport coats, dress pants and shined our shoes. Neither one of us had looked this good since the last Easter Sunday we went to church. We wanted Mr. Freihofer to know he wasn't dealing with a couple of hicks. We drove to Troy in my 1949 black Mercury Hardtop that I polished up the day before. Freihofer's office was next to the new bakery facility. We walked into the fancy mezzanine and told the receptionist that we needed to see Mr. Freihofer and that he was expecting us. The building was brand new and it had that smell about it, new and expensive. The ceiling looked to be mahogany and the walls and floors glistened with white marble tiles. The receptionist asked us to be seated and as we sat down on the plush leather chairs Tommy leaned over and said sarcastically, "Do you still think our white shirts and striped ties will impress him?"

We waited for about thirty minutes and Mr. Freihofer came bounding into the mezzanine. With his hand extended, he welcomed us, "Sorry you had to wait boys, come on back to my office." His office was even more impressive than the reception area.

He sat behind a large antique desk and I commented on how beautiful it was. He proudly told us that the desk had once belonged to the patriot DeWitt Clinton. He began the meeting and said, "So boys, you want to buy the old bakery building. You did a great job in cleaning out the old machinery."

I replied, "Yes sir, we think it will be an excellent place for a nightclub and restaurant, plenty of space and parking."

"I agree but that's a tough business especially in a town like Albany. Just between you and me, one of the reasons I relocated here in Troy was that damn O'Toole machine is so hard to do business with."

Tommy asked, "What do you mean?"

"Well, Uncle Riley O'Toole wants so damn much under the table or he'll find a way to shut you down. You do know about the machine, don't you boys?" He replied.

Of course we knew that the Democratic Party boss Riley O'Toole ran everything in Albany. But there were many successful clubs, bars and restaurants in Albany. They made it work. "We appreciate your advice and we'll definitely look into that." I said, then asked, "Mr. Freihofer, how much do you want for the building?"

He replied, "I'm anxious to sell, so I'm willing to let it go for $50,000, trust me, that's a bargain."

Tommy said, "That sounds fair, can you give us a week or so to talk to our banker and do a little more ground work. Maybe we ought to talk to our alderman, seeing as how you mentioned Riley O'Toole."

"Sure, sure, you do that and by the way if you are going to open a nightclub, you better talk to some of your paisans." He said, looking straight at me.

"What do you mean?" I asked.

He replied, "Well, if you expect to have your garbage picked up or hire any entertainment, or buy whiskey, you're going to have to talk to them."

We got up to leave and Mr. Freihofer shook our hands and said one more thing. "Boys, I'll have to know your intentions in a week. I have one other interested buyer, a church. Some holy-roller church called The New Albany Church of God. They made me an offer but in all honesty, I'd rather not sell to them. My brothers over at the Knights of Columbus Hall might not understand. But business is business. Just be sure to let me know by next week." He concluded.

We left his office and drove back to Albany with plenty to think about. "Tommy," I said, "we need to work on a budget. We need to know what our monthly expenses will be, starting with the mortgage and the equipment loan from State Bank." Then I added, "The New Albany Church of God.... I've heard of that church.... Nevertheless it's not a real church, it's not Catholic."

We agreed that we would see Mr. Birch at the bank together. He said we could come by the next morning. The other tasks we divided between us. Tommy, being Irish, had a better in with the O'Toole machine. He went to see his Alderman, a fellow by the name of Pat Murphy. And I, being Italian, went to see a local wiseguy, a fellow named Mickey King. His real name was Santino Crocetti and he was my uncle. Both our contacts assured us that they would work with us and help us out as much as possible and not to worry about a thing.

For the next week, all we did was work on the club. We didn't take the truck out once for any scrap work. The big thing on our minds was the bank loan. We figured we could handle both the machine and the mob, after all everybody knew us and knew we were stand up guys. Surely, they would work with us just like they said.

Mr. Birch went with us to check out the building. We told him about our plans for the nightclub. We had been very careful to always pay the truck loan on time. He liked the building and thought $50,000 was an excellent price. In fact, he said at that price we would have made $25,000 in equity right from the start. We applied for a $75,000 loan. We would make a down payment of $15,000. We figured that with a loan of $75,000 plus our down payment we could buy the building and have enough for remodeling the interior and all the restaurant equipment we would need. We had another $5,000 set aside to do the initial stocking of alcohol and food and pay the help until we got going. Mr. Birch estimated that our monthly payments over a 10 year period at 4% interest would be $800. That sounded reasonable to us.

The next week we called Mr. Freihofer and told him we wanted to come by his office and make him an offer for the building. He said he would be out of town until Wednesday but we could come by around 10 on Wednesday morning.

That Tuesday before our meeting, my mother called and asked me and Tommy to come by her house after supper. I asked her why she wanted both of us to come but she just said for me to please come by and that it was very important. The invitation seemed strange but Tommy agreed to come with me and we arrived at my mother's at 7. My mother and father lived upstairs over Concino's Bakery on Pearl Street. She always insisted that anyone entering her home remove their shoes and not traipse dirt on to her clean floors. Everyone always obliged and so Tommy and I removed our shoes. As we walked into the living room, we found my Aunt Camille, her husband Charlie and a middle age man that I had never met, who was introduced as Anthony Marcone or Brother Anthony as my mother and Camille called him.

We sat down on my mother's couch that was covered by a clear plastic slip cover. Aunt Camille, who was even more outspoken than my mother began the conversation. "Sonny, we heard that you and Tommy are trying to buy the old Freihofer Bakery building over on Spruce Street."

I replied, "Yes we are. How did you hear about that, have you been talking to Rosie?"

"No, Mr. Jack Freihofer told us. Our church wants to buy the building and we thought we had a deal but Mr. Freihofer told us that he was selling to a man named Sonny Angelo and his friend." Camille explained.

Now I remembered why the New Albany Church of God sounded familiar. It was Camille's church and my mother had just started going there as well.

Brother Anthony then said, "Sonny, we've come to ask you and Tommy to withdraw your bid, to step aside, so that we can buy the building for the new church."

My mother added, "Sonny, we've been meeting in an old warehouse on Green Street. It's a terrible building but at least it was a place to have church. Now the owner says he has a new tenant and we have to be out by next month. Can't you find another building that would work as well for your restaurant?"

"Ma, we'd like to help you out but this building is perfect for our nightclub. This has been our dream to have a place like this and now we actually have the money to make it possible. Don't you see this is a once in a lifetime opportunity." I said, as I looked over at Tommy who was nodding in agreement.

Aunt Camille jumped in and said, "Sonny, if you only knew how much this means to us. Having this building can open so many doors for ministry in this city. I am begging you, not only for God's sake but for your sake...."

I interrupted her saying, "My sake, what do you mean my sake. This is the biggest opportunity of my life. This means that Tommy and I won't have to be in the truck searching for scrap metal at 6 in the morning in freezing weather just to eak out a living. We've both got families we have to support. What could be more important then that? Certainly not some holy roller church." With that I went too far. My mother started to cry. Brother Anthony asked me to please reconsider and Camille said, "Sonny, God cannot bless this adventure of yours. You need to repent and ask Him to forgive you."

"You're not even a real church, you're not Catholic!" I said and got up and motioned for Tommy to follow as I walked out of the room to leave the apartment.

As we left my parents apartment I said, "Tommy can you believe that. We're not giving up our future just so some holy rollers have a place to meet and jump around the place with their hands up in the air. Have you seen that guy Oral Roberts on TV? He's one of them." Tommy agreed and we both started to laugh.

The next day we drove to Troy to meet Jack Freihofer. Once again we wore our best Easter clothes and gave him our offer of $50,000 which he accepted. Two weeks later we met with Jack Freihofer's lawyer at Mr. Birch's office in the bank and closed the deal. We were now the proud owners of "The Bakery", soon to be Albany's newest and most exciting night spot. This was almost too easy.

CHAPTER 15

OUR DREAM COMES TRUE

The next couple of months were probably the most exciting time of my life. We were consumed with all the details of getting the club up and running. Tommy and I made lists of everything that needed to be done and divided the work.

I did my best to rebuild the bridge I had burned with my mother and Aunt Camille. The New Albany Church of God didn't survive. They couldn't find a place to hold their services. The religious culture of the times was not accepting of such a Pentecostal church. My mother went back to St. Anthony's Catholic Church. I considered that good for her. It's where she belonged. My mother was one of the best cooks in Albany and she even agreed to help out some in the kitchen. On the other hand, Aunt Camille said that she was praying for me, that she loved me but what I did was wrong. As a Christian, she said that she forgave me. She ended up driving 45 minutes out to Nassau in Rensselaer County to attend another Pentecostal Church out in the sticks. Because the church was so important to her, she and her husband Charlie moved to a small house in the country close to her new church. I didn't see much of her after that. She blamed me for their former pastor, Brother Anthony, leaving Albany and returning to Buffalo. There just wasn't much call for Pentecostal preachers in a town as Catholic as Albany.

Our carpenter friend, Carlo Crishone, built the stage as well as a beautiful bar. The bar was contemporary in style and made of solid mahogany with brass foot rests, it was beautiful. Across from the bar we built a platform raised about a foot off the floor for our stage. We left plenty of room for a dance floor. "The Bakery" was classy and sophisticated. We took down the old Freihofer sign and replaced it with a big neon sign. It lit up the whole neighborhood. We were able to get all the kitchen equipment from a friend of Mickey King's at a real good price. There was no telling where Mickey's friend got the equipment but it was top of the line and we didn't ask any questions.

While all the madness swirled around us with remodeling the interior of the club, these two big black guys came walking in asking to see the owners. Tommy ran up to them and gruffly said, "Can I help you?"

The older one said, "Yes sir, we heard that you were planning on having live entertainment in your club."

I stepped up and replied, "That's right, why are you asking?"

"Well, me and my brother have a band, the High Life's. My name is Ben McGraw and I play the piano. This is my brother Harold and he plays the bass. Along with us we have two other friends, one is a drummer and the other blows trumpet. We thought we'd come by and see if maybe you were still looking for a house band. We're real good and times being what they are, we'll work cheap." He said.

"Come by tomorrow night about eight and bring your friends and audition for us. If you're any good we'll talk about it." I replied.

I found out that they knew my mother from the New Albany Church of God. I wondered why they didn't mention that. At any rate, we had been talking about a house band before they came in. If they could play, this was another piece of the puzzle falling into place.

Tommy was concerned that an all colored band might be a problem, but I reasoned, "Most of the blacks stay below Pearl Street. I didn't think it would be a problem. As long as they are part of the help, the white customers won't care, that is if they can play." As for me, I was excited to have a band to back me up. The McGraw brothers and their band came by the next night and I must say I was quite impressed. They were excellent musicians and could play jazz and pop and even do some back-up vocals. This was exactly the kind of house band I had envisioned.

As construction on the interior of the club grew close to being completed, we busied ourselves with everything we needed to do for our Grand Opening on May 1st, 1953. Tommy took care of getting the county and city business licenses. We put an ad in the Knickerbocker News for waiters, waitresses, bar tenders, hat check girl, cigarette girl, cooks, busboys and dishwashers. I interviewed all the applicants and hired the help. I hired Johnny Canavi to manage the bar. He promised to behave himself. The wait staff was experienced and I was really impressed by this girl by the name of Judy Tortelli. Recently divorced, she was a real looker and about my age, a real asset to "The Bakery". The gossip was that her ex used to beat her up. I hired a chef away from Lombardo's named Sal Russo. We put him in charge of the kitchen. My mother liked him and Sal told me he was happy to let her help out now and then.

One Friday, Tommy and I drove down to New York City to the Copacabana. We wanted see how one of the best nightclubs in the country ran their business. What a great night. The place was so impressive. We were able to get a table in the far back section of the club. We didn't mind, the club was packed. We were lucky to get in at all. Jerry Vale was the headliner and was someone I really looked up to. He was fantastic. If only we could get him to sing at "The Bakery." As we drove back home to Albany that night, both Tommy and I were so excited. We weren't crazy enough to think "The Bakery" would become the next Copacabana, especially with it being in Albany, but we could see the possibilities.

As the big night for the grand opening approached, everything was coming together. Chef Russo had the kitchen well stocked and was doing an excellent job. I don't know if we could have pulled this off without him. We would specialize, of course, in Italian Cuisine. Because the name of our club was "The Bakery", we thought that it was important that we also be known for our baked desserts. We were lucky enough to find this guy from Sicily, Onofrio Corrcione. The customers loved his specialties, tiramisu, canolis, and ricotta cakes. Under my supervision, Johnny had the bar ready to go. Tommy would be out front greeting the all the first nighters and I would perform with the High Life's. We advertised in the local newspapers, the Times Union and Knickerbocker News, as well as the main radio station in town. We paid a couple of teenage boys to hand out flyers all over downtown. Even the weather forecast was in our favor, calling for a clear and mild night.

The big day was finally here and everybody was busy doing last minute spit and polish work inside the club. It was about four hours before we were set to open, when two guys dressed in dark suits walked into the club. Johnny went up to them and told them we weren't open until 5:30. They told him they needed to see the owner. When Johnny told them I was busy and they needed to make an appointment, things got ugly. Johnny came back to the office looking disturbed and said, "Sonny, we have two guys out there that need to see you."

"Tell them I'm too busy, this is opening night. They'll have to come back Monday." I replied.

"That's what I told them but they insist on seeing you now. They said that if you won't see them, then we won't have an opening night," said Johnny.

"What do they look like?" I asked.

"Serious, very serious." He replied.

Well that got my attention, so I went into the bar area where they were waiting. "Gentlemen, hello, I'm Sonny Angelo. How can I help you?" I asked, trying to lighten up what appeared to be a tense situation.

"We're from the County License Bureau. I don't think your county or city licenses are in order. You need to fix this right now or we're shutting you down." He said, with no emotion in his voice. Johnny was right, they seemed serious.

I told Johnny to find Tommy and tell him that he needed to come up here now and to bring copies of the licenses. I asked to see some identification and they pulled some official looking badges that said Albany County Inspector. Tommy came running to the bar area waiving the licenses. "What's all this about, I went to the court house and filled out the applications and paid the fees. We have the licenses. What's the problem?" Tommy shouted. He was not as diplomatic as I was. That's why we made such a good team.

One the inspectors said, "We sent one of our guys here last week and spoke to your bar manager." He growled, pointing to Johnny Canavi. He continued, "Our guy asked him how many cases of Hedrick's Beer did he want and he said none. You can't open up unless you buy at least 20 cases of Hedrick's every week. It's a license requirement."

Tommy said, "Oh, I see what's going on. Listen boys, I talked to Pat Murphy and he said we were OK."

The man replied, "It's because of Pat Murphy that your order is only 20 cases of beer and not 30."

Hedrick's Brewery was owned by Riley "Uncle Riley" O'Toole. He ran the Democratic Party in Albany and the Democratic Party ran everything else in Albany. Even the mob didn't mess with the Democratic political machine in Albany. I looked at Tommy and then turned to the men and asked. "How much will it take to make our licenses right?"

"Because it was necessary for us to come out today, there's a penalty, this week it's $400. If you pay on time, hereafter it'll be $200. Every Wednesday Hedrick's will deliver 20 cases of beer. Be ready to pay up the $200 right then or your license is cancelled. If you can't pay on Wednesday we'll shut you down. The fee to reinstate your license is $500. So don't be late." He said, with a lot of sarcasm in his voice.

Well that was $400 we hadn't counted on spending but you just didn't mess with the machine. I had Johnny go the cash register and get $400. I handed it over to them. As they turned and began to leave the club, one of them said, "Good luck on your opening, boys….Oh, and enjoy the beer." Both men were laughing as they walked out our front door.

We stood there for a minute just shaking our heads. I guess there was still a lot we had to learn about the club business. I looked at Johnny and fussed at him, "Why didn't you tell me some guy came in here from Hedrick's? You know who owns that brewery!" He just shrugged his shoulders and went behind the bar.

With this problem temporarily solved, our minds raced back to the excitement of opening night. Tommy and I bought brand new suits from Solomon Brothers for the occasion. The wait staff wore white shirts with black cummerbunds, black pants and black bow ties, even the busboys. The hat check girl and cigarette girl wore low cut black cocktail dresses and the High Life's all wore dark colored suits. Regardless of the expense this was going to be a classy joint.

The doors opened at 5:30 and by 8 o'clock the place was packed as I prepared to come out for the opening number. Tommy was the MC and gave me a big introduction. The band began to play, "I've Got the World on a String," and boy, that's the way I felt. I sang for two hours that night with only a 20 minute break and I could have sung all night. The crowd loved it! There were several girls; all in their early twenties, who crowded the stage and screamed when I sang a Sinatra song as if I were the man himself. Fortunately for me and Tommy, our wives were home with the kids. What they don't know won't hurt them, right?

Our Grand Opening wasn't just a one night fluke either. We did great business every night. Chef Sal's food was excellent and we got a Four Star recommendation from the food editor of the Times Union. Onofrio's baked deserts were a big hit. People called for reservations just for the food and we were booked two weeks in advance. On Friday and Saturday nights we had live entertainment and had to turn people away. We did so well that we were able to book some nationally known talent like Julius La Rosa and even the great Joe E. Lewis performed at our club. I actually opened for Joe E. Lewis! Can you believe that?

The cash was really flowing in. I was able to set my father up in his own tailor shop. This was something he had always dreamt of.

Being able to help my father fulfill his dreams; now that was wonderful. My mother divided her time between helping him out in the tailor shop and working in our kitchen. As my father's business grew, she left our kitchen to work in the tailor shop full time. When we were still working the scrap metal business, Rosie and I had planned on buying a house in the country. But now it was important that we live close to "The Bakery." Tommy and I were putting in at least twelve hours every day at the club. I didn't want to be driving a long distance to and from the house. We decided to buy a two story brown stone on Madison Avenue. The house was convenient to the club and had plenty of space and it even had two bathrooms.

Tommy and I were both able to achieve the ultimate in status when we each bought a 1954 Cadillac; shiny black ones at that. One of our friends told us that the boys in Pat's Barber Shop were really buzzing when they saw me drive past the shop in the new car. I finally had some respect. I was no longer the guy who couldn't enlist in the service during the war because of my club foot. I was somebody. It was heaven.

CHAPTER 16

DOWNWARD SPIRAL

Christmas time 1953 was approaching and all continued to go our way. It was just past noon and we were decorating the club for the holiday festivities. We set up a big Christmas tree just inside the entrance way. Judy Tortelli had become our best waitress and she was helping me decorate the tree. She laughed at my method for of adding tinsel to the tree decorations.

"Sonny, you have to put the tinsel on the tree one piece at a time. You don't just throw a ball of tinsel on the tree, silly," she teased.

I guess I knew almost from the time I hired her that she had a little crush on me. "Judy, this gives me the affect I'm after. I know what I'm doing." I flirted back. Just because you're married doesn't mean you can't have some harmless fun. Anyway, you couldn't deny that Judy was real cute, dark hair and eyes and what a figure. I had to admit, married man or not, I was attracted to her.

In the midst of this harmless fun, a man came walking into the club. His face was all too familiar to me. He came walking from the past into my present and I can't say I was happy to see him. David Greene was one of the toughest and most feared men in Albany. He was half Italian and half Jewish and our history went all the way back to school days at Schuyler High. There was an intense incident at the bowling alley between Johnny Canavi and David where I was forced to step in to help Johnny. For reasons unknown except to David, he backed down rather than fight me. I always considered that night one of the luckiest nights of my life. David worked as a collector and enforcer for the local bookies and loan sharks. He also did some free lance work for both the mob and the O'Toole political machine. On top of all that, it was rumored that he had killed several men. I wondered what he was doing here. It wouldn't take long for me to find out.

"Sonny, long time, no see." David said, as he extended his hand in friendship. David wore an expensive suit and looked as though his business, so called, was very successful.

"David Greene, you old son of a gun, good to see you. What brings you to "The Bakery"? What are you drinking?" I asked, putting on my best face but wishing with all my heart that he hadn't walked through the doors.

He replied, "Anisette and a cup of coffee, black, please."

"Judy, sweetheart, be a dear and get us two Anisettes and coffee." Judy must have sensed that this was not a pleasant social visit as she hurried to the bar to bring our drinks as Mike and I found a quiet booth off to the side to talk.

We exchanged small talk while we waited on our drinks. Judy came quickly with the drinks and left us alone. "So David, what brings you here today? Not that I'm not glad to see you, but it has been awhile. I'm sorry that Tommy isn't here. He's out doing some last minute Christmas shopping." I explained.

"Sonny, I have a business proposition for you that I hope you'll seriously consider." He said.

"Business proposition?" I replied.

"This part of town has gotten, how shall I put it, is kinda dangerous. The nice people who come to your club now might stop coming if they thought this area isn't so safe. Well, I can promise you that if you accept my proposal that won't happen. No one will dare rob or harass any of your customers or bother your club. I mean, you won't be in business long if some of these thugs start breaking the club's windows or vandalizing your patron's cars." David explained, as he stared at me without blinking his cold dark eyes. I understood what David was getting at. The best word to describe being in his presence was intimidating.

"David, this is an interesting proposal. But this part of town is safe already. We've had no problems whatsoever. Tommy talked to Pat Murphy and I talked to my uncle Mickey King. We have their blessing and their protection. Maybe you ought to talk to them and see just how safe this neighborhood is." I suggested without backing down.

"Sonny, I've always liked and respected you. Because of that I'll give you until just after New Years to give me your decision. My protection will cost $1,000 each month and I promise you, no one and I do mean no one, will bother you about anything. You and Tommy need to go back and talk to Pat Murphy and Mickey King. Discuss my offer between yourselves and I'll be back right after New Years. I'll expect your answer then." He said, speaking softly but his undertone of menace and intimidation was unmistakable.

David Greene was a man to be taken seriously. I called all over town looking for Tommy. The first thought that came to my mind was that Tommy needed to see Pat Murphy and I needed to visit Mickey King just as David suggested. We'll call his hand and see if he is bluffing. An hour later Tommy came walking through the door whistling some happy little Christmas tune. He was totally unaware of the news I was about to lay on him.

"Tommy, we've got to talk. We have a problem. While you were out we had a visitor, David Greene." I explained.

Having just come in from the cold, Tommy's rosy colored checks began to turn pale white. "What did he want?" He asked, with obvious concern in his voice.

I replied, "He wants $1,000 every month to protect the club."

"This is a shakedown, plain and simple. He'll get a grand a month over my dead body." Stated Tommy defiantly.

"That's kinda what he implied would happen if we didn't agree to his "proposal". For starters I'll go talk to Mickey King and why don't you go to Pat Murphy. Let's see if they can help us." I suggested.

Tommy went to see Pat and I went down to my uncle's candy store. Mickey King's store was on the corner of Herkimer and Green Streets. The candy store was just a front for the gambling operation in the back. It was also the pickup and drop location for the city lottery run by the O'Toole machine. Uncle Mickey knew everyone in Albany. He had what some of the boys downtown called, a lot of "juice." My uncle changed his name back in the 30's when he was hiding from the Genovese Family from New York. At that time he went by his birth name Santino Crocetti. He had an identical twin brother, Carlo, who was not involved at all with the mob. In fact, Carlo worked for Albany Savings Bank and always kept his nose clean. Santino on the other hand would do anything legal or otherwise to make a buck, including stealing from the mob. The Genovese Family found out that Santino kept two sets of books for the numbers racket he ran for the family. You don't steal from Vito Genovese. They sent a couple of hit men up to Albany to make any example of Santino. Unfortunately for Carlo, he was mistaken for his twin brother Santino and murdered by the

Genovese soldiers, gunned down as he was walking to his brother's store. Santino changed his name to Mickey King and disappeared until after the war broke out. Somehow, and we're not sure how, he was able to make peace with the Genovese Family and return to Albany. He liked his new name so much that he kept it.

When I entered the candy store, a fellow named Sammy was working at the front counter. He knew who I was and directed me to the back room. The back room was actually a mini casino with poker and blackjack tables, a craps table and roulette wheel and had a fully stocked bar. As I approached my uncle he hugged and kissed me and asked. "Sonny my boy, it's good to see you, sit down and have some coffee. Now that you're a big shot you don't come around so much anymore." He said with a big grin on his face.

"Uncle Mickey, I need your counsel." I began, "I had a very unpleasant visit from a man I used to know."

He replied, "What's troubling you, who came to see you?"

"Do you know a man by the name of David Greene?" I asked.

"Sonny, this is not good. He's a very bad man. You must take him very seriously." He advised. His face changed from friendly to very concerned.

"That's why I'm here. He wants us to pay him a grand each month for protection. I told him we didn't need protection but he insists we do. I guess this would be protection from him. What do you think?" I asked, hoping Uncle Mickey could call his Patron and make David Greene go away.

"Sonny, it's been all over town that you and Tommy are both driving shiny new black Cadillac's. The word is that you are making a ton of money. What's wrong with you? You set yourself up for this. Never let anyone know if you are doing good or doing bad. This man is like a shark that smells blood." He said, then added, "Go back to your business and I'll find out what's really going on. Give me a few days and I'll let you know what you must do."

I didn't feel much better after my visit to Mickey King. When I arrived back at the club, Tommy was waiting for me. He didn't look very happy. "What did you find out?" Tommy asked, hoping I had found a solution.

"Well, not much, Mickey King is going to make some calls. He'll let me know in a few days if there is a way out of this, short of paying David that money. He thinks we set ourselves up by driving our fancy cars." I reported. Then I asked Tommy, "Was Pat Murphy any help?"

"Pat said that the machine and the mob heard how good we were doing and decided they needed to charge us more for the privilege of doing business. It is Pat's understanding that David was sent by the O'Toole machine. Greene is also connected to some mob big wig from the city. Pat said that there is no way out of this and his advice is to pay the money, shut up and to not mess with David Greene." He replied.

"Between the $200 a month we have to pay for the Hedrick's beer and now this, we'll really have to start watching our expenses, but do we really have a choice?" I said.

Tommy said, "Let's wait and see what your uncle finds out. We'll deal with this after the holidays."

Tommy got up and left and I stayed there sitting in the booth and smoked a cigarette contemplating this sudden turn of events. What if we do pay this "protection money", what's stopping them from coming back and wanting two grand a month? Judy walked up behind the booth as I sat there in obvious distress and began to rub my neck and shoulders. "Sonny, relax, you're so tense. It's going to be all right." She said, trying to comfort me. She always seemed to know exactly what to do.

The next day, Sammy from my uncle's store came to the club with an envelope from Mickey King. I opened the envelope and pulled out a piece of writing paper. On the paper two words were written, "Pay it", signed "MK".

My life was spent in the club. I was there probably 16 hours every day. I was never home. When I did go home, all Rosie did was complain that she and the boys never saw me anymore. She was always mad that I never helped her with the boys. I was so tired of her nagging. I couldn't wait to get back to the club. After all, wasn't I providing a good home for her and the boys? Was it too much to ask for some peace and quiet at home? I felt that the only person that seemed to understand the real me was Judy.

We decided to close the club on Christmas Eve and Christmas Day. Then we would reopen on the 26th and begin to get ready for our big New Years Eve party. We had the whole family, both Rosie's and mine, over to the new house on Christmas Day. I must admit, this was a very happy time. Rosie was in a good mood, for a change, and the boys loved everything that Santa brought them. We took a picture of the three boys dressed up in their new cowboy hats and wearing their guns and holster sets that they just got for Christmas. We had them squat down and look up as I snapped the picture. It was a great day.

When I returned to the club, we prepared to open up for the dinner crowd. I overheard Judy singing. To my surprise, she had a very pretty singing voice. "What's that you're singing?" I asked.

She replied, "Embraceable You by Louis Prima and Keely Smith, do you like it? I think it's new."

"Yeah I do. You have a very good voice. Maybe you and I could sing that as a duet on New Year's Eve." I suggested.

"Well, I've never sung in public before but it has always been sort of a fantasy for me to be a singer. Do you think we could?" She asked.

"Why not, I'll ask Ben and the boys if they know the tune and we can rehearse." I replied.

New Year's Eve arrived and the crowd was as big as we hoped. We charged $35 per person entrance fee and that included the meal and a bottle of champagne. We really needed the business, if we were now forced to pay David Greene a grand a month. The High Life's were in fine form and, if I say so myself, I never sounded better. I could tell Judy was very nervous about our duet and when the time came I made the introduction.

"Ladies and Gentlemen, it is my privilege to introduce you to a little lady who is going to make her singing debut here tonight. Many of you already know her. She has been working at "The Bakery" since we opened our doors. Without further ado, please welcome Judy Tortelli."

The crowd loved the song. We did "Embraceable You" just like Louis and Keely, in fact, I think they would have been proud. Judy had a real bluesy quality to her voice and at one point during the song Ben yelled out, "You sing it, sister!" "Sister" became her nickname and from then on everyone called Judy "sister". At the conclusion of the song, we both sang "embrace me my sweet embraceable you" and as part of the act, we did embrace and look lovingly into each other's eyes. With the sound of applause ringing in our ears, we stood there for a moment still holding each other and suddenly, our embrace was not just part of our performance. Something had happened between us. Sparks flew and my heart began to beat a little faster and my face flushed. I had this funny feeling welling up inside of me. We stepped back and just smiled at each other, both knowing something had happened and both wondering what might lie ahead.

As the clock counted down to midnight and 1953 became 1954, the band played Auld Lang Syne. We had streamers and confetti fall from the ceiling and everyone looked for someone to kiss. I knew it was wrong but I didn't care. I ran off the stage and found Judy. Taking her by the hand, I led her back to my office. We kissed each other passionately. We were both mad for each other. I never wanted a woman so much in my life. Sweeping everything from the top of my desk, we desperately made love right there in my office. I never realized passion quite like this before. It was so surreal, like a beautiful dream. Voices outside my office door brought us back to reality. We quickly straightened our clothes and I asked her to leave the office first. "We'll talk about all this after New Year's Day." I told her.

As she was leaving, she turned and said, "Sonny, I'm in love with you, but you know that don't you?"

I replied, "I do, and I'm in love with you too. What the hell are we going to do?"

CHAPER 17

THE TATTERED WEB

"The Bakery" was closed on New Year's Day and I spent a very tense day at home. All I could think about was Judy and how much I wanted her. Rosie kept asking me, "Sonny, what's wrong with you? What's on your mind?" I made excuses that I was exhausted from the big New Year's Eve we had at the club and I was concerned about having to deal with David Greene. Both of those answers were true but in reality my mind was on Judy, how much I wanted her and just what the hell was I going to do about it. Everything else took a back seat, even my kids. Frankie was having trouble in school and to add to everything else, Rosie told me we had to bring him to school tomorrow and meet with the principal.

January 2, 1954 was the beginning of a rocky new year. Rosie and I brought the kids to school to discuss my 7 year old Frankie's problems. The principal explained that Frankie was a "bit of a handful". Apparently, Frankie was into all kinds of mischief. Among other things he stole money from his teacher's pocketbook, was pushing other kids when they were standing in the lunch line and he even brought matches to school and attempted to start a fire in the cloakroom.

"Mr. Angelo, your son is showing all the signs of a boy crying for attention. If his behavior doesn't improve, I'm afraid we'll have to expel him from school," said Mr. Warner, the principal.

Rosie chimed in, "See Sonny, I told you. Mr. Warner, my husband is never at home and I have two other boys I have to worry about. Tell him he needs to be a better father. These two older boys aren't even mine and their real mother never wants to see them. It has all fallen on me." Rosie started to cry as she poured out her complaints to the principal.

I quickly jumped in and said, "I'll try to be home more but we opened this new business last year and it just takes all my time. I'm trying to build something for my family. What can I do? Isn't my main responsibility to provide for my family?"

Mr. Warner replied. "I understand but I can't help you with any of that. I'm concerned about your boy but my responsibility is for all the kids in this school. You'll just have to find a way to handle this."

Before we left the school, I had a stern talk with Frankie. He just kept nodding his head that he understood, as I warned him of the consequences if he didn't shape up. Tears rolled down his cheeks and he promised to do better.

I dropped Rosie off at the house and headed to the club. As I pulled into "The Bakery's" parking lot, there was Judy sitting in her car waiting for me. I had to resist the urge to grab her right there and kiss her, remembering that someone might see us. I wasn't quite ready to go public with our romance. However, as soon as I unlocked the door and we were away from the front windows, we fell into each other's arms and kissed passionately.

"Sonny, I haven't thought about anything else but you since New Year's Eve," said Judy.

"Baby, I know, I've never felt this way about anyone. I just believe we are supposed to be together but I've got to figure all this out." I said.

Just then Tommy pulled into the parking lot and we had to act as though our love for each other wasn't the most important thing in the world. We pretended to be boss and employee, for now anyway.

Soon the entire staff was in the club cleaning the mess left behind from New Year's Eve and getting ready to open that evening. Despite all my other problems, I could think of nothing else other than how madly in love I was with Judy. Then Tommy brought me back to reality when he said, "Sonny, I guess we can expect a visit from David Greene today. What do you think?"

"He said he'd be here right after New Year's. We put all that money in the night deposit bag. When I go to the bank, I'll get $1,000 in cash and we'll have it ready whenever he shows up." I said.

Just then Johnny Canavi walked by and he overheard part of our conversation. Neither Tommy nor I told him about our visit from David Greene. We knew the bad blood between the two that went back to high school days was still very real. Johnny asked, "What are you two mamalukes talking about? Who might show up?"

I looked at Tommy and knew I had to fill Johnny in on what was going on. Johnny worked for us, that was true enough but he had been our best friend since elementary school. I told Johnny that we were expecting David Greene to show up sometime in the next few days. "Johnny, I know there's bad blood between you two, so when he comes in, do me a favor and just go hang out in the back. Have a smoke or something, OK?" Johnny got this sick look on his face. He had always been a guy who was ready for a fight but he was smart enough to be afraid of David Greene.

We waited for three days. Every time someone walked into the club, I imagined it was David. I thought to myself, where is he already, what's his game? Finally on January 8th, David walked through the door. Fortunately, Johnny was doing stock work in the back and I was able to get Judy off to the side to have her tell Johnny to stay in the back.

"David, how's it going? I hope you had a Merry Christmas." I said extending my hand to him.

He was all business wanting to know my response to his proposal. "Sonny, you've had some time to consider my business proposition. What did you and Tommy decide?"

"Have a seat while I go to my office and get the first installment. Do you want a cup of coffee?" I asked him. I could see his face relax when he knew we had agreed to pay him.

"Very good, very good, you're a smart guy, Sonny. You'll be in business for a long time." He said, as I left to get the envelope with the $1,000 cash.

David was in a hurry. He took the cash and cordially warned that he'd be back next month. Then he was out the door. I hated giving him that much money but I rationalized that this was just the cost of doing business. It was overhead.

That crisis over, I still had to deal with the question of Rosie and Judy. I'd been through a divorce before but that was different. My first wife cheated on me and she was glad that I took the two older boys when I left. Now I had a third boy, Ricardo. If I divorced Rosie, she would take Ricky and leave the two older boys with me. How was I going to handle raising my sons? Would Judy be willing to take on that responsibility?

All I really knew is that I couldn't keep my hands off Judy and Rosie was getting suspicious. Men are terrible liars, when I went home, I had a hard time looking Rosie in the face, let alone touching her in the bedroom. This anxiety continued for a few months. Judy was pressuring me to do something. Several times a week, I would sneak away from work and go to Judy's apartment on Morton Avenue. Our love making was wonderful but it wasn't enough for her. She threatened to quit "The Bakery" and break off our relationship. At home, Rosie had that woman's intuition and it was telling her I was cheating. We fought like cats and dogs. The whole situation was taking a toll on all of us especially the kids.

Then finally, one night I came dragging into the house at two in the morning after being with Judy. Rosie was sitting in the kitchen waiting for me. She'd been crying. "Sonny, tell me who she is."

I knew I couldn't hide this from her any longer so I confessed. "Rosie, honey, I'm sorry. I'm in love with another woman. I didn't mean for this to happen. It just did. I'm sorry."

What's that old expression, "Hell hath no fury", Rosie stood up and slapped me across my face as hard as she could and called me a rotten bastard. I had it coming and she sure deserved better than I gave her. As she stormed out she said, "I'm leaving tomorrow morning with Ricardo. Nothing you can say will change my mind. You'll be hearing from my lawyer." She ran to the bedroom and locked the door.

It hard to imagine but just a few short years before, I fell in love with Rosie. She was just a sweet teenage girl then with a crush on me. I had already been married and divorced and had two kids. We use to hang out at the Waldorf Cafeteria after the dances with our friends. I pretended not to be interested in her but finally gave in after one of her friends told me that she had gotten over me and was interested in this other guy. I guess that stoked my competitive spirit, so I called her and out of the blue proposed to her over the phone. I remember trying to be as charming as possible and singing the song "Pretty Baby" to win her heart. It worked and we were married a month later in Connecticut. Now, it was over between us. The heart is a fickle master. All I knew was that I was in love with Judy.

The next couple of days were rough. My mother came over to help with Bobby and Frankie but her heart wasn't in it. She had always believed that they were not my sons, especially Frankie. Because of her suspicions she never really accepted them as her grandsons. I knew better but she just couldn't love them like she loved Ricardo. I heard that Rosie and Ricardo took a train to New York City and were staying with her aunt. She wanted to be as far away from me as possible. I felt so guilty about Rosie that even my passion for Judy had faded. She could feel that my love had grown cold and she said to me, "Let me know when you decide what you want out of life." She pulled away from me and within a week told me that she was quitting "The Bakery" and that her ex-husband had called and wanted to get back with her. She thought that was the best thing for her right now. Just like that, this woman who I was so sure was the great love of my life was gone. What was I thinking? How could I have screwed up everybody's life like that?

My mother told me that she would look after the boys for another week, but after that I would have to make some other arrangement. She and my father were very busy at the tailor shop. They had expanded and now were selling fine men's clothing and competing with Solomon Brothers. There was no way that I could continue to manage "The Bakery" and be both mother and father for these boys. On top of that I got the divorce papers from Rosie's lawyer and she wanted $600 a month for Alimony and child support. Business had been good but paying David Greene and the Hedrick's people was starting to cut into our profits.

Someone told me about LaSalle Home for Boys in Albany. This was a good place for orphaned boys and boys that came from situations like mine. I just wasn't able to care for them anymore. I was a man not a mother. I tried to give them a home. I deserve credit for that, don't I? Their mother didn't care for them like I did. Anyone could see that.

I went to LaSalle and talked to the Jesuit Brothers. They asked if there was any way that I could help pay the boys expenses. I figured I could give them $200 a month, $100 for each boy. They assured me that they would provide a stable home and a good environment for the boys. So I made arrangements to bring the boys to LaSalle the next day. That night I got the boys together and told them what was going to happen. Both of them started to cry but Frankie was especially upset.

I didn't sleep at all that night and in the morning I tried to get the boys ready. Frankie was screaming. He begged me not to take him away. He cried out that he was sorry for all the bad things he had done and he promised that he'd be good from now on. At one point he grabbed hold of the kitchen table leg and refused to let go. Finally, I was able to get him free and pick him up and forced him into the back seat of my Cadillac. The crying and screaming didn't stop even after we got to LaSalle. The brothers were waiting on us and they picked up Frankie as he was kicking and screaming. Little Bobby went along compliantly. He just had this look of resignation and disappointment on his face. I promised to get them some weekends and that we'd be together soon and have a lot of fun.

I walked to my car relieved that this episode was over. I really meant it when I told them that I would come and get them some weekends and I always meant to. But I had to sing most every Friday and Saturday nights and I was just exhausted on Sunday. I did the best I could. Anyone could see that, right?

CHAPTER 18

RAINY DAYS

S everal months passed by and "The Bakery" was doing alright. We made enough to pay all the bills, pay off David Greene and machine and I still had some left over to live and be on time with my alimony checks. However, emotionally I was on shaky ground. Losing Rosie and the boys and then to have Judy leave me was more than I could handle. Sure, there were several girls who would hang around the stage after my performance but that was only a temporary diversion. With my broken heart on my sleeve, I went down to Herkimer Street and spent some time with my Uncle Peter and his wife Estelle. This was my old neighborhood and everybody knew me. There I was sitting on the stoop of Peter's apartment and suddenly I burst into tears. The events of the past several months came welling up inside of me. It was June in Albany and everyone was outside sitting on their own stoop. I started to sob even louder. Peter, although he was my uncle, was actually only a few months older than me. He was embarrassed by this spectacle, "Sonny, for heaven's sake, please stop crying!" He begged. But I wouldn't. Many of the neighbors came over and offered their comfort and concern. I needed the sympathy. Peter told me I made a fool of myself. Maybe I did, but letting this all out made me feel much better.

David Greene would always come by the club between the first and third of the month to collect his grand. So far we were fortunate that the club was doing well enough that this wasn't a problem. We were careful to try to keep Johnny Canavi out of sight when David arrived, no sense in asking for trouble. Then on the 30th of June, out of the blue, David Greene came walking into the club. This was a few days earlier than usual and we didn't expect him. Johnny was cleaning near the entrance and looked up when he heard the door open and suddenly he was face to face with his old nemesis.

"Well, well, I thought this place had some class. I guess I was wrong, if they let a low down dog deserter like you work here."

David said very sarcastically. David Greene, as bad a man as he was, served honorably as a Marine in the Pacific Theatre. He was on Iwo Jima. It was well known that Johnny also joined the Marines but couldn't handle the discipline and went AWOL. He spent most of the war in federal prison.

Johnny was never one to back down if confronted even from someone like David Greene. He was very sensitive about being labeled a deserter. As he explained it to me, fear of going off to war had nothing to do with him going AWOL. It was that damn drill sergeant always in his face. After David insulted him, Johnny stood right in front of him and shouted, "Greene, you go to hell!"

David started to laugh at him and said, "You're probably right about that. That's where I'm going and I'll see you down there. Now go get your boss and tell him I'm here!"

Fortunately, I heard Johnny shouting and immediately came out of my office to see what was going on. I quickly intervened and told Johnny to go in the back and have a smoke. Walking up to David, I extended my hand. Normally he was friendly enough but now he refused the offer of a handshake. "David, I didn't expect you today. You're early." I said.

"I'm going down to New York City for the 4th of July to meet with a friend of my father's. This guy is a very important man and I want to get this stuff out of the way. I'll be leaving first thing in the morning and won't have time for this tomorrow. Do you have my money?" He demanded.

"David, not right this minute. We haven't gone to the bank today. We were planning to have it for you tomorrow. All our cash is in the night deposit at the bank or in our accounts. We have some of it here but not all." I explained.

"Go to the bank today and get it. I've got some other business to take care of and I'll be back around closing time. Have it ready for me then." He said and then started to leave but stopped as if he remembered something else. "Sonny, I always figured you for a smart guy. Letting a bum like Johnny Canavi work for you, that's not so smart." With that said, he was out the door.

I walked into the kitchen and there was Johnny. He had been listening to my conversation with David Greene.

"Sonny, why do you let that guy talk to you like that? And where does he get off calling me a bum. I've hated him since 9th grade." Complained Johnny.

I replied, "Johnny, I don't like him either but if you are going to be in this business, you just have to play ball with these guys."

About that time Tommy came in and I explained that David Greene wanted the money early. "Tommy, I have this bad feeling, I think we both need to be here when David Greene comes for the money. Neither one of us should be alone with him. I don't know why, but I just have this feeling in my gut." Tommy agreed and also thought that Johnny should leave work early. We didn't want him around stirring the pot.

As always, we put ten $100 bills in an envelope to pay for our monthly "protection". As Tommy suggested, Johnny was sent home early. It was mid week and it had been raining off and on all night, so it was a slow night. We closed early and sent everyone home. Tommy and I sat at the bar and had a drink while we waited for David Greene. We were both tired and getting irritated as it was almost one o'clock in the morning and still no David. Finally, at fifteen minutes past one we saw headlights shining into our glass entrance as his car pulled into the parking lot.

David Greene walked in and it was obvious that he had been drinking. He was extra abusive and sarcastic. "Where's my money? C'mon, I don't have all night." He blurted.

I walked behind the bar and opened the cash register and retrieved the envelope with the cash. Then David said, "Because you guys are so stupid, stupid enough to hire that bum Johnny Canavi, I want an extra $500."

"David, be reasonable. We can barely make this payment and we certainly aren't ready to pay that tonight." I said.

"Bullshit! Let me see what's in that till." He slurred and started to go around the bar.

Tommy was fed up. He stood in David's way blocking him from going around the bar to the cash register. David Greene was one bad man but Tommy at 300 lbs wasn't a pushover either. David must have made a mental decision that in his half drunk state even he was no match for a relatively sober Tommy Phelan. David stepped back and reached inside his jacket and pulled out his gun. He pointed it at Tommy and warned him, "Move out of the way or die!"

Tommy froze and just stared at David's gun. I yelled, "Tommy, it's not worth it, just move!" Tommy still stood there as if it hadn't registered in his brain that a .38 caliber hand gun was pointing at him. David smiled and said, "You know what, I'm going to enjoy this." He cocked the trigger and raised the gun to Tommy's eye level.

Suddenly, Johnny came out of the shadows running toward David with a baseball bat. David was taken completely by surprise and didn't know what hit him as Johnny swung the bat at his head with all his might. David dropped to the floor like a sack of potatoes. Johnny, relieving years of pent up hatred for him, kept bashing David's head with the bat. I ran over and jumped on Johnny knocking him to the floor to stop him. David's face was unrecognizable. Blood was splattered everywhere. Tommy was still standing behind the bar with David's blood all over him. I went over to David. He wasn't breathing. He was dead, Johnny killed him.

"Johnny, man, look what you just did!" I shouted.

"I just saved your ass, that's what I just did! He was about to drop the hammer on Tommy. Do you think he would have let you live once he shot Tommy? You were next. I had to do it. That louse had it coming!" Johnny shouted back.

Johnny hadn't gone home after we closed the club. He had planned to jump David Greene in the parking lot because of the stuff David said to him earlier that day about being a deserter. As an ex-con, Johnny wasn't allowed to own a gun so he always carried a baseball bat in his car for protection. This bat was one of his prize possessions. Johnny dropped out of school when he was 16 years old, after his old man threw him out of his house. The next year our baseball team at Schuyler High won the city baseball championship. Each team member got a championship bat with the inscription, "Schuyler High School 1941 Albany City Champs." I felt really bad that Johnny couldn't play that year so I gave him my bat.

After he left the club, instead of going home, he parked his car a few buildings up on Spruce Street where he could watch the club parking lot. When he saw David pull in, he walked up to the entrance of the club and was going to wait for David to leave. "I was going to take his legs out with the bat as he walked to the parking lot. I looked inside the club from the glass door and could see that David pulled his gun. With all the commotion, I guess you guys didn't hear me come in. Once I was inside I knew I had to act quickly or we were all going to die here tonight." Johnny explained, as he gasped for air, he couldn't calm down.

My mind started to race, understanding that our lives were in extreme danger. Trying to remain calm I said, "We don't have time to talk about what happened or why it happened. Our problem now is how to get rid of the body. We need to dispose of David's car and get ourselves and this place cleaned up. I don't know if the machine or the mob will understand why Johnny killed one of their own."

We picked up David's gun and took our envelope with the ten $100 bills. We found his car keys and wallet then we wrapped his body in a couple of table cloths. We were careful to remove anything that could identify him as David Greene including his ring and watch. Tommy and I carried his body out to the parking lot and put him in the trunk of his Lincoln. We searched the car for anything that could identify it as belonging to David. All we found was a bag with eleven envelopes full of cash. Apparently, we were David's last stop of the night. We took the envelopes and left the bag. We counted the money and there was $15,000 in cash in those envelopes. We decided that we would split the money three ways.

I was always good at figuring things out but never thought I would need that ability for something like this. "Boys, here is what we're going to do. Johnny, here's his car keys. Do you know that small dump on Catherine Street?" I questioned.

"The one near Swan Street?" Johnny replied.

"Yeah, that's the one. There's nothing over there and no gate to keep us out. Drive the body to that dump. Tommy and I will follow in my car. We'll bury his body under the garbage. The rats will do the rest. After we do that, we'll drive down to the Hudson River Scrap Yard. They keep the fence chained at night but we've got some chain cutters in the utility room in the back. Abe Sokol always leaves the keys in the forklift and shredder. We can lift David's Lincoln with the forklift and drop it into the shredder. I've seen that shedder squish a car down to the size of a bread box." I explained, as they nodded in agreement.

People were always spilling drinks and tomato sauce on the floor, so we had plenty of industrial strength cleaner in the supply closet. It took us about an hour to clean the area. I made Tommy and Johnny take off their clothes and go back to the locker room and put on whatever they could find that fit. I did the same. We always had clean cook's and waiter uniforms back there. We took our bloody clothes and threw them into the trunk with David's body. It started raining again. I would have rather burned the clothes at the dump. But the rain would make that impossible. I figured that we could just scatter them under the garbage. We had some rubber gloves in the kitchen that the cooks sometimes used. I made everyone wear a pair. We didn't want our finger prints on anything.

It was now three o'clock in the morning and we had less than three hours to get all this done. We made it to the Catherine Street dump in about fifteen minutes. I was careful to park on the street so there would be no tire tracks and no mud on my car. I had always been an avid reader of Erle Stanley Gardner and had read enough Perry Mason novels to know that it was the little details criminals overlooked that did them in. Johnny drove the Lincoln right up to the edge of the dump. We quickly got out of my car and ran up to him. Johnny held the flash light and carried two shovels as Tommy and I lifted David Greene's body out of the trunk. We carried the body about 100 yards into the dump site until we found a suitably disgusting place to bury the body. The place stunk to high heaven. Because of the rain we had to slog through mud, making the situation that much more miserable and nasty. We cut up all of our blood soaked clothing and scattered the pieces about, putting them under some garbage to discourage any dump divers. Then we randomly threw David's ring, watch and wallet deep into the dump. We had carefully removed all David's identification and cut it up in small pieces before scattering that. We kept his gun and planned on shredding it at the scrap yard.

It was four o'clock and the only thing left to do was to go to the scrap yard. Johnny drove the Lincoln with me and Tommy following. Driving up to Swan Street, we cut over to Morton Avenue and went all the way south until Morton Avenue turned into Rensselaer Street. Then we drove the short distance to the scrap yard on the Hudson River. As we pulled up to the gate, we turned our head lights off and got out of the car. We parked behind David's Lincoln. It started to rain even harder. From my point of view this was a good thing. It meant nobody was out, especially at four in the morning in a rain storm. Even the police wouldn't be out on patrol. The downside of the rain was that we were all drenched making our work more difficult.

Just as we thought, the gate was chained so Tommy took the cutters out as I held the flashlight for him and he broke the lock. We pulled both cars into the scrap yard so they were out of sight. Tommy and I had been in this yard many times and had even operated the forklift and shredder when Abe Sokol's work got backed up, so we knew what we were doing. On those occasions, Abe would give us an additional five cents per pound of scrap. We drove the Lincoln up close to the shredder. Fortunately, the scrap yard was all paved with gravel so at least we didn't have to contend with the mud again. Tommy ran to the forklift and as we hoped, Abe had left the keys in the ignition. Before lifting the car into the shredder, I removed the license plates. Using the chain cutter, I cut the plates into several small pieces and then threw them onto different heaps of scrap metal around the yard. Tommy fired up the forklift and drove it into position sliding the forks underneath the car. I turned the shredder on. Tommy lifted the Lincoln into position and luckily dropped it right into the shredder on the first try. The shredder made mince meat out of that car. In a matter of minutes the car was in thousands of pieces piled up in a small mound. I can't imagine anyone ever tracing David's car. While the shredder was still running we threw David's gun in as well.

Abe Sokol obviously would know that someone broke into the yard because of the cut lock. After returning the forklift to its original spot we wanted to disguise our true reason for breaking into the yard. So we broke into Abe's office to make it look as though we came into the yard to burglarize his office. With that done, the three of us got into my car and drove back to the club. It was now 5:15 AM. Abe usually got to the yard around 5:30, so we really cut it close. To the best of my knowledge, no one saw us.

When we got back to the club we vowed that no matter what, none of us would ever talk about this night or implicate each other and no matter what, we would all deny any involvement in David Greene's death and the cover up. I was very concerned about the $15,000 cash. If people saw us spreading around a lot of dough it might raise suspicions. I wanted to burn the cash but was overruled by Tommy and Johnny.

"Look, the reason we had to pay for 'protection' in the first place was because we started driving the Cadillac's. I don't want to die over 15 grand." I reasoned. Finally, we each agreed to keep $500 for now and put the rest in the safe. If it seemed reasonable to do so, we could split the money later, maybe in a year or so.

We agreed that the story we would stick to if anyone ever asked was this. David Greene came by the club in the afternoon on June 30th and he wanted us to pay $1,000 right then. I told him that we weren't expecting him and I didn't have the money ready and would have to go to the bank. He said that he had some other business and would come back around closing time to pick up the money. He mentioned that he was going to the City in the morning and wanted to get this out of the way. Tommy and I were closing the club and were by ourselves when David came in around 1:15 in the morning. He had been drinking and it appeared that he had one too many. All that was true up to that point. Then we would swear that after we gave David the envelope with the cash, he left and drove away and we haven't seen him since. Johnny was to always say that he wasn't at the club because we sent him home early as it was a slow night on account of the rain.

Three days later the trauma of that night was just starting to fade when Mickey King and a couple of scary looking guys walked into the club just as we were opening for dinner. My heart went into my throat as I rushed to the lobby to greet them.

"Uncle Mickey, it's so good to see you. Do you and your friends want a table for dinner? Your money's no good here, everything is on the house." I said, embracing my uncle kissing him on the cheek.

"Sonny, how have you been, you never come to see me anymore." He said and looking at one of the other guys, "My sister's son is a big shot now. He never comes to see his uncle. You oughta hear this boy sing, better than Sinatra, I swear." Then turning back to me he said, "Sonny, have you seen David Greene lately?"

I got this sick feeling in my stomach as the two guys with my uncle looked me over searching for some reaction. "Uncle Mickey, we saw David two, maybe three days ago. It was the day before July 1st. I remember because he came a day early for the money. Usually he would come on the first of the month." I went through the story just like we planned it. Yes we saw him, he left with the money and that's all we know.

Then I asked, "What's up with David. Like I said he had been drinking a lot."

He replied, "We don't know. He made about a dozen collections that day but he never turned the money in. People all over the east coast are looking for him. We'll give you credit for this month because your story jives with everything else we heard but starting next month, Paulie here, will be by on the first, so be ready, capisci."

I replied, "I understand, no problem."

They didn't seem suspicious. This was great. They thought that David took the collection money and bolted. We were home free. As for David Greene, well as Johnny said, "That louse had it coming."

Later that night, just as I was going to bed something hit me. The baseball bat, what happened to the bat? Did we throw it into the trunk with David's body? The next day I asked Tommy and Johnny if they remembered what we did with the bat. Tommy thought we dropped it in the trunk of David's car with the body but Johnny thought we threw the bat into the Catherine Street dump. Nobody could agree on what became of the bat. I thought our cover up was iron tight. Over the years I would wake up in a cold sweat worrying about that bat.

CHAPTER 19

THE BEVERLY HILLS CLUB

Weeks turned into months then years and we realized that as long as we all kept our mouths shut no one could tie us to David Greene's death. In my mind, I never thought of what happened that rainy night as murder. If there was ever a case of self defense, this was it. David would have wasted all of us. I'm sure of that. We had to cover this up. The wise guys wouldn't care if it was self defense. We killed one of their own and their rules say someone has to pay. It was the way they protected themselves.

It was now 1958 and "The Bakery" was doing pretty good. We had a steady clientele, a group of regulars that would come in every week no matter what. On weekends we provided solid entertainment with me and the High Life's and every month we featured a nationally known celebrity. So what if we never got Frank Sinatra or Dean Martin, our customers was still excited to see singers like Vaughn Monroe, Eartha Kitt and comedians like Jan Murray and Totie Fields. We were just this small club in Albany and these entertainers had worked Las Vegas.

On the downside, Tommy was slipping a bit. He had developed a pretty bad drinking problem. He started drinking when he got to the club at about 11:00 AM and usually drank steadily until closing. I'll give him this; he could really hold his booze. The way he was living his life was taking a toll on his family. Before we opened the club, family was just about the most important thing in his life. Now, between his drinking and whoring around, he hardly ever saw his wife and four kids. I'm not one to talk. I averaged seeing my kids maybe twice a year. At least I provided for them. There is something to be said for that.

Ben McGraw was a heck of a piano player and for a musician making his living playing in a saloon, he was very reliable. He never missed a gig. So, we were very concerned on Friday when Ben was a no-show. I sat in on keyboards and did a passable job but nowhere near the ability of Ben. Ben's brother Harold left as soon as our last set was over to try to find out about him.

The next day Harold called to tell me that Ben was in critical condition at Albany Medical Center. He said, "Mr. Sonny, Ben is in bad shape. They beat him so hard they almost killed him."

"Is he going to be alright? Who beat him?" I asked.

"The police did and the doctors don't know if he's going to make it." Harold sobbed.

Apparently, Ben was walking down Madison Avenue and happened upon a white man and woman in a heated argument. The man backhanded the woman and Ben intervened to help her. Just then a cop pulled up to investigate the fracas. The white man accused Ben of attacking them. His woman was too intimidated and abused to disagree and tell the cop the truth. The cop started to swing his Billy Club landing a couple of blows to Ben's head. By now another cop was on the scene and he joined in by kicking and stomping Ben. Ben was a gentle soul and was just trying to help a woman but for his trouble he was beaten to within an inch of his life.

Tommy and I were all too familiar with these loose cannons that were given a badge, a gun and all the authority to satisfy a very bad attitude. Years before when we were still in the scrap business, we would go out to the sticks in Rensselaer County. Our rule was, if we saw anything that contained metal such as old junk cars, washing machines, hot water heaters or farm equipment and it was within twenty feet of the road, even if it was behind a fence, then it was junk and could be scrapped. We couldn't help it if the property owner was not available to confirm that it was junk. We'd just take it and if we could lift or dismantle it, it went on the truck. Was it stealing? We justified taking it by saying no it wasn't. After all, if the owner wanted it, then he should have taken better care of the property. One day, unfortunately for us, Tommy and I were in the process of taking some "junk" from behind a fence on a lonely country road. Two Rensselaer County Deputy Sheriffs came riding by. Pulling their guns, they had us get on the ground. They frisked and then handcuffed us and threw us to get into the back of their patrol car.

We thought that we would end up in prison for grand theft as the "junk" we were dismantling was a working tractor owned by a local farmer. They drove to a county substation and directed us into a cell inside the building. We tried to convince them that we thought the tractor was just scrap metal and we would gladly pay for any damage. We waited in the cell for two hours. Finally, they came and got us and we went back into the patrol car. They drove down an old unmarked dirt road. I noticed that a second Sheriff's patrol car was following. We stopped and they ordered us out of the car. Our hands were still cuffed behind our backs. Two other deputies stepped out of the second patrol car. They told us that this is what will happen to anyone who comes into Rensselaer County to steal scrap. They warned us, "Be sure you tell all your friends about this!" The four deputies proceeded to beat the living daylights out of us. Both Tommy and I were knocked unconscious. When we woke up, we were lying in the middle of the road next to our truck. Our faces were a bloody mess. We could barely get up and walk to the truck. For good measure the cops busted out the head and tail lights on the truck. Somehow we made it home. Neither Tommy nor I was able to work for over a week.

The police in upstate New York did whatever they felt necessary to uphold the law, even if it meant breaking the law. As for poor Ben, it was months before he was able to get outside and walk or drive a car. Several of his fingers had been stomped on and were broken. He once had such a beautiful fluid style to his piano playing. Well, that was gone. His nerves were shot and he was just a shell of his old self. Ben became a very bitter man. Apparently, there were some other witnesses who were willing to come forward and vouch for Ben. Because of this, all charges were dropped and of course no charges were ever filed against the police officers who brutally beat Ben. There were two kinds of justice in Albany, New York, one kind for white people and the other for black people. Maybe someday the police won't just assume the black man is guilty. Maybe someday they'll bother to ask questions first before swinging their Billy Club at someone's head.

As for the High Life's, the week after Ben was beaten, the band broke up. He was the heart of the group. They weren't any good without him. "The Bakery" was now without a house band and unable to provide live music on weekends. This band is what made "The Bakery" so special. We auditioned several other combos and some of them weren't half bad but they were not the High Life's. Some of our regulars stopped coming in and business started to fall off. As we moved into 1959 we started to hurt for money. The rest of the $15,000 we took from David Greene that we stashed in the safe was long gone.

I went to see my uncle, Mickey King and explained our problem. "Uncle Mickey, things are getting tight for me and Tommy. I don't think we can keep on paying the $1,000 a month for "protection" and the $200 for Hedrick's Beer and keep our doors open. Is there anything you can do to help us?"

My uncle said he would make some calls and get back to me in a day or so. "Sonny, there may be some other way that will keep the boys happy and still let you keep the business open. I'll see. Wait for my call."

Two days later Mickey King and two associates came by "The Bakery" to discuss business. Tommy and I led our guests to a private both in the rear of the club. One of the men, Tony Rizzi, did most of the talking. My uncle and the other man were careful to always call him Mr. Rizzi. He said he had just come up from Jersey and might be interested in helping us out.

"Mickey says that your business is off and you need a little help making your bills." Mr. Rizzi said.

I explained to Mr. Rizzi how our business had suffered after the breakup of the High Life's. If we could just have some relief from our monthly payments and also a small loan to bring in some well known entertainers, I was sure we could get back on our feet.

Mr. Rizzi then said, "I'm not a banker, you need a loan, go to a bank. However, I might be interested in becoming a partner, investing in your club."

Tommy blurted out, "No offense Mr. Rizzi, but if you became our partner, who'd be calling the shots?"

"Boys, you've tried it your way and where did it get you. If you don't do something, you lose the club and end up with nothing. I'm offering you an opportunity to at least have something." He explained.

I replied, "Tommy, I think we should at least listen to Mr. Rizzi." I said, motioning for Mr. Rizzi to make his proposal.

"You guys will have to be flexible. We have to change the business and make it into a private club. No more food, it loses money, only booze, it makes money. We'll make this into a casino. We're very friendly with the local political machine. I've already spoken to them and they're on board. We'll cut them in for a nice percentage and they'll provide the legal protection. Now, of course my guys will run the operation. They know what they are doing. I've checked your records and both of you are clean, so we'll leave the business in your names. All you have to do is show up a few times each week and make appearances here and there when we tell you and you can pick up five grand per month." He said.

"Mr. Rizzi, I'd like a few minutes to discuss this with Tommy, if that's Ok." I said.

Mr. Rizzi, nodded his approval and Tommy and I went into the kitchen and out the back door to talk in private. Five thousand dollars a month was a lot of money and we didn't have many options. It meant giving up our dream. This establishment that we had been so proud of would no longer be ours. As hard as it was, it was the only thing we could do. We went back into the club and sat down across from the three men.

"Mr. Rizzi, Tommy and I discussed this and we accept your generous offer." I said.

The three men all flashed smiles and my uncle Mickey said, "Bravo Sonny, congratulations!"

Mr. Rizzi said that we had to close "The Bakery" by the end of the week. He said to pay whatever we could to the staff as severance and put a sign on the door "closed for renovations." They would send people up from Jersey to renovate the club just the way they wanted it. The last thing Mr. Rizzi said was, "When we reopen, I don't want to see your little friend Johnny Canavi coming around here. Word is; he's got a big mouth. Be sure you take care of that, first thing. I heard some bad things about him from an old friend of mine."

The hardest thing we had to do was to tell the employees we were closing. Not having to pay the $1,000 in protection money gave us a little extra to pay the staff. Johnny however, was not too happy. We tried to reason with him and even tried to give him a little extra money but the way he saw it, we were telling him that our lifelong friendship was over. I don't know what he did to be in Dutch with the mob but if Mr. Rizzi expressly said to be sure Johnny doesn't come around, then it was best for everyone if Johnny stayed away.

Three months later the new club was ready for its grand opening night. On the roof of the building the new sign beamed in neon "The Beverly Hills Club." Most of the windows were bricked or changed to opaque stained glass making it impossible for anyone outside the club to look in. Inside, our once massive dance floor now provided ample space for all sorts of gaming tables, card tables, crap tables and a large roulette wheel. Along one wall glistened a dozen slot machines and next to that wall, several cashiers sat behind glass enclosures to exchange money for chips. Then there was the crowning jewel of the club, the bar. The custom made mahogany bar was extended making it 100 feet in length. A special form of gambling was embedded into the bar itself. At the bar, before each club member seat, there was a circle of numbers resembling a roulette wheel. A corresponding roulette wheel was displayed in the center of the bar area. On the wall located above the roulette wheel was a nude figure of a woman named "Lady Luck." Every hour the Lady Luck Roulette wheel would spin and the patron whose circle of numbers flashed would win a shower of silver dollars falling from the nude's hands. The Beverly Hills Club was really something.

Tommy and I wore tuxedos and acted as greeters for the new club members. Each club member paid a $25 membership fee and was given a Golden Beverly Hills Club Card that allowed them entrance for future visits. The place was open 24 hours a day and always packed. Tommy and I got paid but speaking for myself, it broke my heart. Albany was the state capital and several state assemblymen and senators showed up for the opening and thereafter would be frequent guests of the club. Women, of let's say, questionable virtue, were always at the club to entertain the patrons especially the senators and assemblymen. Among other things, they hustled drinks and really increased the club's gross. Bags of money would be dropped off and picked up at regular intervals. I knew not to ask questions. All Tommy and I needed to do was show up, smile and keep our mouths shut.

We never saw Johnny Canavi. From time to time we would hear rumors that someone saw him at a local bar or at the track up at Saratoga in August. We regretted treating him like that but we had no choice. We would be forever bound by our youth and by the terrible night we spent in the rain. The bottom line, we had to do what we had to do.

CHAPTER 20

HEARTBREAK

It was 1960 and Tommy and I had it pretty good. The Beverly Hills Club did great business, we did whatever Mr. Rizzi told us and we always got paid. But life always has its ups and downs. There are good times and bad times, I guess this is the natural order of things. But what happened as the year progressed was not natural.

One night I received a call from Ben McGraw. I hadn't heard from him in a long while. "Mr. Frank, can you come and bail me out of jail?" He had gotten drunk and unruly and the police arrested him. Apparently, Ben's life had taken a real downward turn after he was beaten so badly by the police. No longer able to play the piano with anywhere near his former ability, he was now an alcoholic and extremely bitter about his life. His brother Harold was so disgusted with him that he wouldn't bail his brother out of jail. The only other person Ben could think to call was me. His wife left him a year ago and took their kids. She wouldn't stay with a man who couldn't hold a job and was drunk half the time.

I drove down to the Albany County jail, paid $50 and got Ben out of jail. I remembered the good guy that played the piano so well. The sweet man that would do anything for you. Oh how he had changed. The police sergeant led Ben out from the cell area into the lobby where I was waiting. He was rail thin, smelled terrible and looked twenty years older than when I last saw him. He must have seen the shock on my face as he apologized for his appearance. "Mr. Frank, I know how bad I look but I've been sick. That's why I drink so much. It's the only thing that gets me through the day," he explained.

I told him not to worry about it but encouraged him that he needed to start taking better care of himself. I drove Ben to a rundown building on Green Street. An old friend of his was letting him sleep in the back. We sat in the car and talked for awhile and he reminded me of the first time we met. "Do you remember me telling you that I knew your mother? I had just started to go to her church, you know, the New Albany Church of God. I sure liked that pastor. I think his name was Brother Anthony. Anyways, that's where I met your mother. She was real nice to me. I hope she's doing OK. It was just about the time when we auditioned for you that the church stopped having services. I always thought that things might have been different for me, you know, better, if that church had stayed open."

I nodded that I understood but didn't want to go into what really happened to the New Albany Church of God. I didn't tell him that my decision to take the Freihofer building was the reason the church closed. Anyway, I gave Ben ten dollars and then we said good bye as Ben got out of the car.

Two days later Harold McGraw called to tell me that the fellow who owned the building where his brother was staying found Ben dead in that back room. He hung himself with his belt. There was an empty bottle of gin on the floor below his feet. That was a sad day. At one time, Ben McGraw was as good as any piano player in the county, as good as Errol Garner, George Shearing, any of them. It was indeed a sad day. Tommy and I went in together and bought Ben a headstone. There was a small graveside service at Albany Rural Cemetery. Ben's status as a veteran enabled Harold to get him a plot in the soldiers section of the cemetery.

As we stood at the graveside during the service, I was surprised by a tap on my shoulder. Turning around I couldn't believe my eyes. It was Judy Tortelli. She had always liked Ben very much. I think we'll always remember that New Year's Eve night when we sang "Embraceable You" and Ben called out to her, "Sing it, Sister."

After the service, Tommy left, he had another appointment but Judy and I went to a local diner in Menands to have a cup of coffee and catch up. I must confess, I still thought about her from time to time. Judy told me that she had left her husband for good about a year ago and that he had already remarried. She finally had enough of the beatings, physical and mental.

"Sonny, you always knew how to treat me like a lady. I think we were both confused back then. Our timing was just off." She said.

Taking this as an invitation I asked, "Have you ever thought about us getting back together? Do you ever think about me?"

She smiled and said, "Yeah, I do. I think about you all the time."

I still had my house on Madison Avenue and asked if she had the time and wanted to come over. She said she did, so she followed me back to my place. I know that coming straight from a funeral usually isn't the best time to make love but we did. It was one of the most satisfying experiences of my life.

Within a month, Judy had moved in and we were living together. Life was good. Under the arrangement with Mr. Rizzi, I was making plenty of money and the hours I was needed at The Beverly Hills Club were reasonable so I was able to spend time with her. Judy quit her job at the Miss Albany Diner and always had a hot meal waiting for me when I got home.

One evening I came home and found Judy sitting at the kitchen table reading this big fancy Bible. "What do have there? What are you reading?" I asked.

"Sonny, this nice man came by today selling theses family Bibles. I hope you don't mind but I put a $10 deposit down. The man said I could examine the Bible for a week and he'd come back and if I didn't like it, he'd give me my money back no questions asked." She explained.

"Honey, I told you never to let a salesman in the house." I complained. "How much will this Bible cost if we keep it?"

She replied. "$125, is that too much? But if you'll just look at it you'll see the quality. It will be something we'll have forever and we can pay it off in monthly installments over three months."

"Why do you need a Bible anyway? We never read the Bible when I was growing up. The priests never told us we needed to read the Bible. No, I'm sorry, that's too much money. When that snake oil salesman shows up, give him the Bible back and be sure to get the $10 deposit." I told her.

She persisted, "Sonny, I love you and I know we got it pretty good but there is just something missing in my life. I think I'm supposed to do more with my life."

"And you think you can find it in that book? Why, you're starting to sound like my crazy Aunt Camille. Do you want to start speaking gibberish like she does?" I said, rolling my eyes to show my sarcasm.

"How is having this book going to hurt anything?" She questioned.

"I'm sorry, my decision is final! Give the book back! Get the deposit back!" I shouted, as I walked out of the kitchen.

Judy didn't speak to me the rest of the night. I guess I hurt her feelings but she was wrong. $125 is a lot of money. The next week Mr. Rizzi asked me and Tommy to go to the track with him up at

Saratoga. Mr. Rizzi had some business at the track and wanted to get up there by 1:30 PM, about an hour before the bugle call to post. For some reason he loved the call to post. He said he found it exciting. Tommy had some other business he had to handle and said he'd be there by the first race. I asked Judy to come and ride with me and Mr. Rizzi. She loved Saratoga and I thought it might be a good way to make amends for our fight over the Bible. Mr. Rizzi said for us to bring the girls if we wanted.

Saratoga in August is special place and a real fun time. I always made it a point to go to the track a couple of times during the season. Mr. Rizzi was in a great mood and I enjoyed our drive from Albany. We arrived at the track right on time and went to the clubhouse where Mr. Rizzi met with an associate from Buffalo. He wanted to speak privately with his friend and asked if Judy and I wouldn't mind grabbing a bite to eat. He said he would catch up with us before the post time. True to his word he did and we reviewed the racing sheets before placing our bets for the first race. About thirty minutes later, Tommy arrived with his date. It turns out the business Tommy had to take care of was picking up this girl named Peggy, who he met at the Beverly Hills Club last week. Tommy's wife had given up trying to check on him and resolved that as long as she had a roof over her head and the kids were provided for, then she wouldn't rock the boat. Mr. Rizzi loved to have people around him, especially pretty women. He was delighted when Tommy and the girl arrived.

Judy really enjoyed the afternoon, even her icy attitude toward me warmed up. When her horse came in first in the 5th race she hugged my neck and gave me a big kiss. However, by the last race Judy began to complain that she had bad stomach cramps maybe it was the food or the drinks and all the excitement. I told Mr. Rizzi that I probably needed to drive Judy home because she wasn't feeling well. However, he really wanted to see the harness races that evening and he wanted me to stay, saying he needed to talk to me about an interesting opportunity that came up earlier in the day when he met with his associate from Buffalo.

Tommy needed to get his girlfriend Peggy back to Albany. Peggy, who was divorced, had young children and needed to relieve the babysitter. So Tommy said he would take Judy home as well. She didn't mind driving back with Tommy, so problem solved.

When the harness races concluded I drove back to Albany with Mr. Rizzi. He told me that he thought I was doing a good job at the Beverly Hills Club and wanted me to open another club in Buffalo.

"Sonny, I like your organizational skills, your way with people. You do a good job at the club but you've got to be tougher with some of these dead beats. They tell me that you've held back the muscle on a few guys that couldn't pay their debts. You have a reputation as being too soft. If you're going to run these clubs for me you have to be heartless. It's business." He lectured.

"Yes sir, I understand. I was a singer and night club guy. I'm still learning the ropes." I explained

Mr. Rizzi laid it all out for me. He said I would be in for a percentage of the gross for both clubs. His plan was that I would be given more responsibility at the Beverly Hills Club over the next ninety days. "Sonny, this will be your audition. You're a singer. You should be used to auditions, right." He said with a laugh.

Mr. Rizzi said that he chose me over Tommy because he didn't like how much Tommy drank. "I don't mind a guy that drinks. But not all the time. It affects your judgment too much. I like Tommy, don't get me wrong but even today, did you see how many he had?"

Mr. Rizzi's driver dropped me off at the house. It was about one o'clock in the morning. The house was dark, no lights on. I thought that was odd. Even if Judy had gone on to bed, she always at least left the kitchen lights on for me. I went to the bedroom and started to panic. Judy wasn't in bed. I ran through the house thinking maybe she passed out because of being sick but she was not in the house. I immediately called Tommy's house. The phone rang several times before his wife answered. She sounded as though she was half asleep.

"Katie, this is Sonny. Put Tommy on." I said, trying to remain calm.

"Sonny, what time is it? Let me check. I don't think he's come home yet." She said. She dropped the phone on the table and went to see if he was anywhere in the house. She came back in a minute and said, "Sonny, he's not here. Why don't you call his girlfriend?" With that, she hung up.

I was frantic with worry. Deep in the pit of my stomach I imagined the worse possible circumstances. I racked my brain trying to remember Tommy's girlfriend's name. It was Peggy something. I had no idea how to get in touch with her. I ran out of the house and jumped into my car and sped off to the club. Maybe Judy was feeling better on the way back from Saratoga and they decided to go to the Beverly Hills Club. I didn't know what to do other than to check that out. When I got to the club, no one had seen Tommy or Judy all night. I was thinking the worse, maybe there was an accident. They left five hours before me and Mr. Rizzi. They might have been involved in an accident and by the time we came through on the way back to town, the accident would have been cleared.

I knew the sergeant at the desk at the South Station Precinct. His name was Billy Thompson. I called him from the phone at the bar. I thought that maybe he could check on any accidents from here to Saratoga. "Hey Billy, it's Sonny, I'm looking for Tommy. We were at the track today and he left about five o'clock this afternoon. Nobody's seen him and I'm really worried about him. I thought maybe you could…."

Billy interrupted me. He sounded kinda sick as he said, "Sonny, you don't know what happened? Tommy was killed last night on the highway. We don't know what went wrong but he ended up crossing over into the northbound lane and hit head on with a semi. I am so sorry you had to find out like this." He said.

I was stunned. What he just told me took my breath away. All was silent for a moment until Billy asked me if I was OK. I came to my senses and a bolt of fear shot through me. What about Judy? Somehow I managed to speak, "Billy, there were two women with him. Do you know about them?" I asked, desperately praying to God Judy was somehow alright.

"I'm sorry. Both women are dead as well. I'm so sorry. Were they friends of yours?" He asked.

I couldn't respond, I just dropped the phone and walked outside. I fell to the ground and sat on the curb outside the club and began to sob. I just lost my best friend and the love of my life in one night. Somewhere I read that a lot of college kids were saying there is no God. Well, for me that was true.

We buried Tommy and Judy on the same day. I was in a daze. I had hoped that just maybe Johnny Canavi would show up for Tommy's funeral but he didn't. It would have been good to see him. He won't forgive us. I knew he was in town. People would tell me they saw him at the track or said he was playing the numbers. We should have stood up for him to Mr. Rizzi. We didn't have the balls.

I bought a headstone for Judy. On it I had written, "My Beloved Judy, The Love of My Life." Her name was carved into the stone, "Judy 'Sister' Tortelli." She always liked that nick name. I asked a friend of mine in the jewelry business to make a gold chain necklace with a gold locket. I had him engrave the words, "My Sweet Embraceable You." The week after the funeral I went back out to the cemetery and fastened that necklace to her headstone. My life will never be the same without her and Tommy.

CHAPTER 21

CAMELOT

After the loss of Judy and Tommy, I felt as though there was nothing left to live for. Yes, I still had three kids but I never saw them. It was as if I didn't know them. I had only myself to blame for that. I loved my boys. I mean they were my kids. But I just didn't have the desire to be part of their lives.

The day that Judy and Tommy died, Mr. Rizzi offered me the opportunity to take over The Beverly Hills Club and also open a new club in Buffalo. His only concern was that I wasn't hard enough. Well, after the accident, I just didn't care anymore. If I still had a heart, it was a cold heart. Mr. Rizzi told me he would let me audition for the job. Before they died, I don't know if I could have been cold enough. Now I was like ice.

I started spending all my time at the club. I only went home to sleep, other than that I was at work. It seemed as though there was nothing left to live for so I lost myself in work. The club and making money became my god. The first thing I did was to ban all employees from gambling. I suspected that at least a few of the employees had been stealing chips and then cashing them in. Employees found with chips in their possession would be fired. We beefed up the security cameras and let everyone know that stealing would be dealt with harshly. Even with all this, one of the blackjack dealers tried to rip us off. His name was Peter Jordan and he had a buddy of his come in the club and sit at his table. One of our floor managers caught Jordan dealing from the bottom of the deck. His buddy was winning big. The floor manager, Phil, came to my office and told me what was going on. I got a couple of the security guys and me and Phil went out and confronted the thieves.

There were a few players sitting at Peter's table along with his accomplice. "Sorry folks, this will be the last hand at this table for an hour or so." I said quietly, so as not to alarm the patrons. A waitress was passing by and I directed her to get the players, we were running off, whatever they were drinking on the house.

"Sonny, what's up?" Asked Peter, with a guilty look on his face.

Peter's buddy started to get up and follow the other players, but I had security block his way. "Will you two gentlemen follow us please? I have something I want to discuss with you." I said, as I led the way through the kitchen and down a flight of stairs to the storage room.

Peter knew he had been caught and as soon as we reached the storage room he began to beg for mercy. "Sonny, please, I'll pay everything back with interest. It really wasn't that much, I swear." His friend just stood there looking sick, not knowing what to expect.

"Peter, I thought you were a stand up guy but we caught you stealing. Now, I'm a nice guy but Mr. Rizzi, well, he hates crooks."

"Please Mr. Angelo, have mercy. Please forgive me! I'll do anything." He begged, falling on his knees. At this point, Peter's buddy started to cry.

Looking at these two lousy SOB's I said. "Sorry, no can do, fellas." Then turning to the muscle, I told them, "Boys, show them what happens to people who try to steal from Mr. Rizzi."

The guys that Mr. Rizzi hired to provide security were big tough men who were very good at their work and enjoyed doing it. They beat the crap out of Peter and his accomplice, what a bloody mess they were. There's no telling how many broken bones they had. I let the beatings go on for about five minutes. "OK boys, they've had enough. Now, drag them upstairs and throw them outside in the back with the rest of the garbage. Call the police and tell them we found these two guys and it looks like they've been mugged. Let the police take care of them." We dumped a bucket of dirty mop water on their heads to revive them. Then I warned Peter and his buddy, "If you guys don't want more of the same or worse, keep your mouths shut. You know you had it coming."

Mr. Rizzi was impressed with the way I had handled the situation. He said I passed the audition. A week later we went to Buffalo to meet with the same man Mr. Rizzi was with that day at the Saratoga track. His name was Freddie Randaccio also known as "The Wolf." He was a capo in the Magaddino Crime Family and rumored to be in line to take over when old man Stefano Magaddino retired. He and Mr. Rizzi were old friends and had been looking for a project to work as partners. With the success of the Beverly Hills Club,

Mr. Randaccio thought opening a similar club could be quite profitable. At Mr. Rizzi's recommendation, Mr. Randaccio was willing to talk to me about running the Buffalo club. Having one of his own to oversee the operation gave Mr. Rizzi confidence that his investment would be more secure. The Buffalo family was affectionately called "The Arm" by the locals. They would take care of paying off the Buffalo police and politicians. "The Arm" would also provide most of the employees and in house security.

We found a suitable location in Buffalo and renovated a vacant factory just like we did in Albany. It was perfect, with plenty of space and lots of parking. By the time the club was ready to open, it was May 1961. The Broadway play Camelot was all the rage, in fact the newspapers had taken to calling President Kennedy's administration, Camelot, comparing it to King Arthur's court. So naturally we called the new club, The Camelot Club. The inside of the club was done up like a medieval castle. It was real classy. In addition to the usual casino gambling, the club became the center for one of the largest bookmaking operations in the eastern half of the country. By the end of 1961 the club was amazingly successful. Cash was pouring in. I kicked butt when I needed to and ran a very tight ship. This made my bosses very happy and I reaped the rewards of that success. I personally made over $1 million that year.

For several years I went back and forth from Albany and Buffalo overseeing both clubs. We were profitable and I watched the books religiously to be sure every penny was accounted for and the bosses received exactly what they had coming. I had great favor with both Mr. Rizzi and Mr. Randaccio and I knew better than to cross them.

The FBI had been turning up the heat on "The Arm" and the other New York crime families. Mr. Randaccio suggested that a meeting of the top bosses from New York City to Chicago would be a good idea. Buffalo was centrally located and would be a logical host for such a meeting. He wanted to discuss family security and ways to combat the Federal Crime Commission and the FBI, who he always referred to as the "Friggin' Bunch of Idiots." Mr. Randaccio and Mr. Rizzi agreed that The Camelot Club would be perfect for the meeting. Years before, in 1957, another such crime summit took place. In their arrogance, the family bosses agreed on a country estate in the small New York town of Apalachin. Over 100 bosses came to the meeting, all driving their big black limos and Cadillac's. They stuck out like sore thumbs. The authorities were alerted that something unusual was coming down at this estate. The FBI raided the place, arresting many of the bosses and for the first time, exposing crime families as being organized. The meeting at The Camelot Club would be different. The club would be closed for a special "Bachelor Party" and indeed there would be a stag party. By agreement, everyone would arrive in nothing flashier than a Buick.

This was quite a feather in my cap that such a prestigious meeting would be held in a club I managed. As for my staff, they were personally warned by me not to discuss this event with anyone, especially their wives and husbands. It was all very hush-hush. There was only one problem. An FBI informant had worked his way into the New Jersey family and reported that something big was coming down at the Camelot Club in Buffalo.

The day of the meeting started off well. All the bosses arrived as scheduled and were quite impressed with the club and the preparations we made for the meeting. Mr. Rizzi proudly introduced me to several of the top bosses as his protégé'. Then all of a sudden we received a phone call from one of our guys in the Buffalo PD that we were about to be raided. It was too late, the building was surrounded. Everyone was arrested and questioned. Several of us, including me, were arrested for illegal gambling. Our lawyers were able to get the charges dropped. However the FBI got a lot of names and some information they could use in their war on crime.

The FBI snitch was found out and killed for his trouble and I was not blamed for what the newspapers referred to as "The Little Apalachin Raid." Even so, The Camelot Club was now on the FBI radar and the police protection we had enjoyed for almost seven years was gone. Within a few months we were forced to close up. I went back to Albany. No matter, I had made a ton of money and quite frankly it was getting to be a drag going to and from Albany and Buffalo. When I think of those years in Buffalo, I'm reminded of a line from the Broadway play;

> "Don't let it be forgot
> That once there was a spot,
> For one brief shining moment
> That was known as Camelot"

CHAPTER 22

WALLS OF SALVATION

While the world in the 1960's was spinning out of control, I was just cruising along. I discovered that without the constraints of a conscience, I was very adept at running the day to day business of "The Beverly Hills Club." Kicking butt came a lot easier, now that I didn't really care about what anyone thought of me. I no longer loved my work. I just did it well and made very good money doing it. All I cared about was keeping Mr. Rizzi happy. Every other month I had a new girlfriend, and this helped ease the boredom of life. I saw my kids from time to time but even that was more out of obligation than anything. My two older sons, Bobby and Frankie, would hint that they sure would love to live with me. When that subject came up I always made some excuse about being too busy. I would usually pull a few $20 bills from my wallet and give it to them. I don't know if I really had a conscience any longer but throwing a couple bills at my kids did make me feel better. I remember hearing that someone in the Bible talked about how everything in life was meaningless. As 1970 approached and I was about to turn 44, I could relate to that, for me life was meaningless.

My mother and father continued to work in their men's clothing shop six days every week. They didn't know anything else and the shop did quite well. The only time I would see my parents was on holidays and occasionally I'd go to the store to visit them. They would never acknowledge what I did for a living. I'm sure they knew I ran an illegal gambling house but refused to discuss it. It was obvious that they didn't approve of my line of work. If asked, they would always say that I was in the restaurant business.

I rarely saw or heard from any of the rest of the family. My Uncle Mickey King passed away a few years back. He had been my source of much of the family news. I heard that the former pastor at the New Albany Church of God, Brother Anthony, had returned to the area and was now the new pastor at my Aunt Camille's church in Nassau. After he moved back, he called my mother and invited her to attend services at the church. She told me that she was going to church with Aunt Camille but it was difficult for her to go all the way out in the country to Nassau.

My Uncle Peter would drive her to church and started to attend the services himself. He actually got religion and joined the church. This was amazing to me because Peter had become a bit of a wild man. His youngest child, a son, had cerebral palsy and died several years earlier. The death of his son changed him. He started to drink heavily and chase women. His wife left him. But now they tell me he's a different man because of Jesus. All I can say to that is, we'll see. My mother called me several times asking me to drive her to church and she would always end up saying, "It would be wonderful if you could stay for the service. I think you would enjoy it. Even your Uncle Peter is going to my church now." I wasn't having any of that. I saw what went on in their services on TV with that Oral Roberts fellow. I always made up an excuse and she always continued to call and ask me to go.

One evening I was in my office at the club going over the books, when I received a call from Aunt Camille. "Sonny, come quick! Your father has been trying to reach you. Your mother collapsed at the store. They think it's her heart. She's at Albany Medical Center, please hurry!"

I dropped everything, ran out of the club and got into my car. I was at the hospital within 15 minutes. As I found my way to her room, my father was sitting just outside. He was so upset and had been crying.

"Pa, how is she? Is she going to be alright?" I asked.

"Sonny, it's not good. She's in a coma. The doctor doesn't think her chances are very good." He said, as tears rolled down his face.

I looked into her hospital room and could see Aunt Camille and a man who I remembered as Brother Anthony saying prayers over her. I asked my father why the priest wasn't here. He told me that she wanted Brother Anthony. I waited until they finished praying and then went into the room. I sat by the bed and held my mother's hand. She was the one person in my life that I cared the most for. This life had beaten most of the emotion out of me but I must confess I still had deep feelings for my mother. I tried to pray but the words just wouldn't come.

Brother Anthony and Aunt Camille waited outside the room with my father. After sitting with my mother for about thirty minutes, I went outside to check on my father. Aunt Camille walked over and put her hand on my shoulder and said, "Sonny, you're mother said to me just last week that if anything ever happened to her she wanted me and Brother Anthony to talk to you about where she's going."

"Where she's going? What do you mean?" I asked. Thinking they might be talking about a nursing home.

"If it is her time, she will be going home to be with the Lord. The word of God tells us that our time here in this body is very brief. Psalm 39 says: 'Let me know how fleeting is my life. You have made my days a mere handbreadth; the span of my years is as nothing before you. Each man's life is but a breath.' Sonny, don't you think it is time for you to change your life, to repent and accept the Lord. Your mother has accepted Jesus and it is her deepest hope that you will also." Camille said.

Brother Anthony quickly stepped in and added. "It doesn't matter what sins you have committed. Jesus offers forgiveness. In fact, Jesus said that he 'did not come to call the righteous but sinners.' The Bible is clear that we are all sinners but there is forgiveness of sins no matter what. Sin must be forgiven or judged. Jesus paid the penalty for your sins on the cross. He did the hard part, now all you have to do is accept his free gift of salvation. Don't think for one minute that your sins are too great to be forgiven. Take David for example, he was an adulterer and a murderer and yet God called David 'a man after my own heart.' Sonny, make your mother's wish come true, open your heart to Jesus." He urged.

They were really coming on strong but I wasn't buying it. However, for my mother's sake I listened politely. I thought to myself that if I wanted my sins forgiven, I'd go to a priest. Then, as they waited for some reaction or a response from me, I said, "Thank you for your concern but I'm a Catholic. You know that. Even so, based on my life and some of the things I've seen and been through, I sometimes question if there really is a God." I said, being brutally honest.

Brother Anthony wasn't ready to give up. He had one more salvo to fire at me. "Sonny, I believe that there is something called 'The Walls of Salvation.' Walls can either offer protection or they can keep you out. Depending on the condition of your heart, the Walls of Salvation either protect you from our enemy, Satan, and all the pitfalls he places before us. Or they can keep you away from the Lord Jesus and God's protection, His blessings and love. Make no mistake, Satan is very real and he'll give you many reasons and excuses not to open your heart to Jesus. He'll try desperately to keep you away from Jesus and the truth. Satan will build his walls so high that no one can climb over them. However with God nothing is impossible, no wall is too high that it can keep those he has called from him. Once you get on God's side of the wall, he'll never forsake you, he'll never lose you. Sonny, won't you pray with us right here and now to accept Jesus and reject your sinful life?"

I will admit I was impressed by his commitment and sincerity. I could see why some people like Camille would be drawn into this religion thing, but not me. I said to Brother Anthony, "I'm sorry but not here and not now." I stood up and walked back into my mother's room to check on her.

My mother hung on for two more days and finally her heart gave out. During that period both Aunt Camille and Brother Anthony stayed with her the whole time. On a number of occasions they prayed in her hospital room and I could hear them mention my name. I didn't care that they were praying for my soul but they were just wasting their breath.

Three days later we buried my mother at Graceland Cemetery. I have to admit I was impressed that almost all of the members of Aunt Camille's church attended the funeral. There was something to be said for that. After the service, Brother Anthony invited me to come to his church any time. "Sonny, you're always welcome and if you just need somebody to talk to, please call me. I hope I'll hear from you." I smiled and politely nodded, knowing I would never step foot in that church. But he did mean well, I'll give him that.

I wondered how my father would survive without Mom. I feared that he wouldn't last long without her. Indeed three months later, I received a concerned phone call from this fellow who worked at my father's store. "Mr. Sonny, your father hasn't come to the store today. It's not like him to be late or at least not to call in. You know how hard he always works." He said.

I went to my father's apartment and found him. He had died in his sleep. I guess you can't ask for a better way to go. We buried him next to my mother. Soon after, I sold his store. Pa was 88 when he died and Mom was 85. Another chapter in life was closed.

CHAPTER 23

GUILTY

1974 brought changes that none of us expected but I guess we should have seen coming. "Uncle Riley" O'Toole, the Democratic Party Chairman, was well into his 80's. His son-in-law, the mayor, was pushing 70. They were both slipping a bit. The people of Albany were getting tired of the corrupt politics-as-usual that had ruled the local government for over 50 years. Change was definitely in the wind. It started when a young upstart Republican attorney, David Goldberg, shocked the county by winning the race for District Attorney. He ran on a pledge to clean up government and unlike most politicians, he actually meant it. He was a true believer.

Mr. Rizzi and I were concerned that the police and political protection "The Beverly Hills Club" had enjoyed for so long was about to be taken away. Our people in the police department told us that District Attorney Goldberg was leaning hard on them to enforce the law. We doubled our payments to the cops and to the now fading Democratic political machine and gained a little time but it was no use. Our days were numbered. Mr. Rizzi knew that police raids, led by the new DA, were imminent. He didn't want to be associated with the club if arrests were going to be made. By the end of 1975, Mr. Rizzi told me to let everyone go and close down "The Beverly Hills Club." We could no longer operate in the open as we had in the past. Up until then, Mr. Rizzi had always been very cordial to me. In fact, I always felt that we had a strong relationship. All of a sudden things seemed different, there was no warmth and he was all business. Mr. Rizzi returned to New York City and I didn't hear from him again. Very soon after, "The Beverly Hills Club" closed for good. The building went up for sale. I was now unemployed. The one saving grace was that I had been able to put back a good bit of money over the years and could retire if I wanted.

One morning I was having coffee and reading my paper at the World's Fair Diner on Madison Avenue. I heard someone call my name. I looked up and to my amazement there was Johnny Canavi. "Sonny, the guys at Pat's Barber Shop told me I might find you here." He said, as he stretched out his hand to shake mine.

I was stunned, "Johnny, I can't believe it. I'm so glad to see you."

"Sonny, I was sorry to hear about Tommy and Judy. I almost came to the funeral but I felt really uncomfortable. I've been thinking about calling you for years but never got up the nerve. Then the other day I ran into your son Ricardo. That made me think that it's been too long and we needed to make peace. I know you had no choice and had to let me go all those years ago. I just thought you and Tommy didn't fight hard enough for me." Johnny said.

I replied, "I've gone over that situation a hundred times in my mind. If I had it to do over again, would I have done it differently, could I? That was a very tough time for us. We were broke. We didn't have a lot of options. But in hindsight, you're right. We should have fought harder for you. Anyway, you're here now and I am truly glad to see you."

Johnny and I spent the next hour catching up. The word on the street was that Johnny had lost a lot of money to a local bookie. Johnny always liked to bet on sports, especially baseball. He always said it made the games more enjoyable. I wondered if this chance meeting was no accident and maybe Johnny thought he could touch me up for a quick loan. I didn't bring this subject up and neither did he. As for me, without the responsibility of the club and with nothing else to do, I had time to reflect a little more on my life. I was delighted to see my old childhood friend. The one subject that neither one of us mentioned was David Greene and that night in the rain. The incident had never been very far from my mind. Every once in awhile, David's name would be mentioned. People always wondered what happened to him. I was surprised to learn that Mr. Rizzi had been a friend of David's.

One day when someone said something about David Greene, Mr. Rizzi gave us his opinion of what became of him. "Everyone thinks that David just took off with all that protection money. I don't think so. David Greene was a hard man to be sure, but he would have never screwed us, not over... what $15,000, $20,000 in cash? No, someone knew he was carrying a lot of cash and they killed him for the money. I'll say this. David was one tough son of a bitch. Whoever it was, either got very lucky or knew what they were doing to get the jump on David Greene. He'd be hard to kill."

I remembered that Mickey King was there that day and he chimed in. "Mr. Rizzi, if you're right and someone killed David Greene, they were pros. His body and his car never turned up."

Mr. Rizzi replied, "I'm betting that David's body is still in that car and is sitting at the bottom of the Hudson River. I promised David's old man that if I ever found out who killed his son, I see that louse dead."

Over the years, anytime the subject of David Greene came up, I tried to leave the room. It made me so uncomfortable, I was afraid I looked guilty. Everyone knew I was one of the last people to see David and I always suspected that people thought I must have been involved in his disappearance.

A few days after our reunion at the World's Fair Diner, I received a call from Johnny, "Hey Sonny, how about you and me going to dinner tonight. Do some more catching up. Whatdya say?"

"Sounds good, where do you want to eat." I replied.

"There's a little place down on Madison Avenue close to Pearl Street called Al's Full Moon Restaurant. I know the brothers who own the place, great Italian food. I haven't been there in a while. Why don't you pick me up at my place? My car is in the shop. How does seven o'clock sound?" Johnny suggested.

Johnny hadn't changed. He was always obsessive about his cars and had them in the shop all the time. I knew the place he was talking about. He was right. Al's was a great place to eat. You could get some of the best Italian food in the city there. I was really looking forward to reminiscing with my old friend and enjoying some excellent food and wine.

Johnny lived on Elm Street, right next to Cathedral Academy. With school being closed for the evening, I was able to park right in front of Johnny's house. Walking up the stoop, I rang Johnny's doorbell. Almost immediately, Johnny answered the door. He was still in his t-shirt. "Sonny, I appreciate you coming to pick me up. I'm not quite ready, come in and sit at the kitchen table while I finish dressing." He said.

I followed Johnny from the entrance down a dimly lit hall that led to his kitchen. As soon as I entered the kitchen, two goons grabbed me and threw me to the ground. They started to beat the crap out me. All I remember was screaming, "Johnny! What the hell is going on! Why!" Then I passed out.

I don't know how long I was out, but when I woke up I was sitting on an old kitchen chair in Johnny's cellar with my hands tied behind the back of the chair. My feet were bound by a rope that was also wrapped around the legs of the chair. The voices of several men surrounded me. The cellar was dimly lit by a single light bulb loosely hanging from the ceiling on an electrical cord. Someone must have bumped their head on the light because it was swinging back and forth. As the light swung, the men would fade in and out of the shadows. I remember thinking that they looked like demons. The cellar was completely below grade with no windows and no outside light. The floor was dirt and that added to the damp musty smell. I felt like I was in hell. They had beaten me pretty good. Blood was flowing into my left eye and from my nose down into my throat. I think my nose was broken making it difficult for me to breathe. As I ran my tongue around my mouth, I could feel that several of my teeth had been knock out or broken. I began to pass out again and imagined my mother was telling me to smile big so she could see my pretty teeth. My ribs felt like they were broken. They must have been kicking me. When I tried to move, my body was racked with pain.

Out of the shadows stepped Mr. Rizzi. I was shocked to see him. It was difficult for me to speak. There was no strength in my voice. I could barely speak above a whisper but I choked out, "Mr. Rizzi, why?"

"Sonny, your friend Johnny Canavi told us an interesting story about a rainy night back in July 1954." Now I understood what was going on. Johnny, that bum, told them about David Greene. He set me up.

Mr. Rizzi continued. "Johnny owes us a lot of money and he couldn't pay. He told us that he had some information to trade us for clearing his account. Apparently, your friend Tommy didn't know how to keep his mouth shut when he was drinking. He spilled the beans to Johnny one night when he was especially drunk. Seems like David Greene came to your club to collect our money. But you didn't want to pay it. David came by at closing time just like he said he would. You sent everyone home, including Johnny Canavi. You hid behind the bar and when Tommy distracted David, you snuck up behind him and hit him over the head with a baseball bat. Then you proceeded to hit David over and over again until he was dead. Not only did you save the grand you owed us but you stole the other fifteen grand David had already collected."

I started to cry, my voice barely audible, "No, no, no, that's not what happened! Please Mr. Rizzi, let me explain. Johnny killed David Greene, I swear to God!"

"Sonny, you snake, we're not stupid. Everyone knows that you sent Johnny home early. You even told your uncle, Mickey King, that when David Greene came by that night it was just you and Tommy at the club. But now you say Johnny did it. What a snake, trying to blame someone else," sneered Mr. Rizzi.

With all my might I coughed out the words, "I'm innocent, I swear to God! Please believe me and have mercy!"

Mr. Rizzi walked slowly around the chair and laughed, "Innocent you say. Then explain this." He said, as he held out his hand. I could just barely see Johnny walk into the dim light and hand Mr. Rizzi a bat. "Sonny, do you know what this is?" I shook my head yes, as tears mixed with my blood flowed down my face. He continued. "Let me read the inscription on this bat, 'Schuyler High School 1941 Albany City Champs'. You played on that team, didn't you Sonny? This is your bat, isn't it? Johnny, he wasn't on that team. He quit school. We searched your office and found the bat hidden behind a cabinet. The damn thing still had David Greene's blood stains on it. What kind of louse keeps something like this? Was this your trophy, Mr. Champ?"

All I could get out in my defense was, "No, no, no! Johnny planted the bat. I gave him that bat. It was his bat!"

Mr. Rizzi looked at me in disgust, "How could I have been so wrong about you. I treated you like a son. That's how I felt about David. The reason David Greene was collecting the protection money early was he was coming to New York to see me. And now I have someone I'd like you to meet."

An older man came forward and stood next to Mr. Rizzi. "Sonny, do you know who this is? This man, one of my oldest and dearest friends, is David's father, Mr. Sol Greene. Now let me tell you what you did to him. You let the world believe that David was a drunk, a cheat and a thief. You stood by and let everyone think that David Greene stole the protection money and then skipped town. Mr. Sol and I knew that could never be true, but you brought dishonor to my good friend's name."

The older man stepped up and grabbing my hair, lifted up my head and spit in my face. Mr. Rizzi began to speak, "Sonny, it's time for you to pay for what you did, a life for a life. We're going to kill you with the same bat you used to kill David." Then he motioned for Johnny to come forward. Mr. Rizzi handed him the bat.

Johnny moved closer and off to the left and prepared to swing. Before he did he said, "Sonny, you deserve this."

Through the blood in my eyes I could see him rear back to swing the bat at my head. The moment seemed to freeze. All the terrible things of my life, all my sins, paraded across my mind. My guilt seemed to bubble over and I found myself thinking, "Yes I do deserve this." For stealing and cheating in the scrap business, I am guilty. For all my pride and self centeredness, I am guilty. For showing no concern for my mother's church, I am guilty. For taking the Freihofer building and turning it into a nightclub and a gambling hall when it could have been a place of worship, I am guilty. For cheating on my wife, I am guilty. For quitting as a father, I am guilty. For caring more about my convenience than spending time with my sons, I am guilty. For covering up a murder, I am guilty. For being ruthless in my business dealings, I am guilty. For all the lives that were ruined in my gambling hall, I am guilty. For all the good I could have done but didn't do, I am guilty. When God sent Brother Anthony back into my life with yet another offer to accept Jesus, I again refused, I am guilty. Right now as the moment of my death is at hand, all the charges of all my sins have been leveled against me and I have been found guilty!

I failed to even attempt to scale the Walls of Salvation. Brother Anthony was right. Walls are built to protect you or to keep you out. I failed miserably in life. I was satisfied to stay on the wrong side of those walls and didn't care to find what is true and meaningful. I settled for what this world has to offer. My natural desire to be selfish and to satisfy my own needs dominated my life and I didn't care about those around me. Now I must pay the penalty for my sins, when I could have accepted Jesus. He paid the price. If only I had said, "Yes, Jesus come into my heart!"

I watched as Johnny drew back, knowing that in a moment the bat would strike my head and send me to death. A vision of an hourglass, the grains of sand pouring out, flashed before me. In a voice that was audible only to my mind I cried out, "Jesus save me!"

I came to consciousness on the other side gasping for air and still crying, "Jesus, save me!" Suddenly, I realized that I was back in my room at the nursing home. Tears of joy filled my eyes. So what if I had MS. So what if I was completely paralyzed. What did it matter, I had Jesus and all was well. I was on the right side of the Walls of Salvation away from all the evil that might have been and God would always protect me. I recalled that dream of so many years ago. The forest, the small cottage and the old priest. He was a messenger from God. My hourglass was now turned right side up. The grains of sand slowly poured to the bottom, almost empty now.

PART III

WHAT WILL BE

CHAPTER 24

A NEW DAY

I lay there on my bed contemplating all that I just saw. I was horrified by what might have been. Indeed, I am a stupid man, a foolish man. For several hours, that sinful life, the other side of me, passed through my mind. Suddenly, my eyes grew weak and I lost my ability to see. Just as suddenly, I was surrounded by brilliant light, more brilliant than the sunniest summer day at the beach. I recalled the previous time that this sensation seized me and still I was filled with fear. The presence of God was with me and began to speak, not audibly but to my mind. I began to pray, "Please Lord, do not send me back!"

The Lord began to speak, "Frank, my son, do not be afraid. You will not be going back to that sinful nature. Around you I have built up the Walls of Salvation which the enemy cannot breach. Do you know about my servant Job?" Asked the Lord.

I replied, "Yes Lord, I know his story well and have read his book many times."

"Satan asked to have Job put into his hands. I knew my servant Job, just as I know all my servants. I granted Satan's request and turned Job over to him. Everything Job had was taken from him. His wealth, his family and his health, all gone. Everything was gone except his very life. But Job did not sin. Like you, he questioned but he did not curse me. I will never put more of a burden on my servants than they are able to carry. In your case, Satan requested that I also place you into his evil hands. The life you might have had would have been the result. Your burden, the illness you bear, was my shield given to you to quench Satan's fiery arrows. From the world's view you have lost everything but from my view you have gained eternity." Said the Lord.

"My Lord and my God, I was weak when I questioned my life. Now that you have shown me what my life would have been, I can only praise you and repeat the words of Job when he said, 'Surely I spoke of things I did not understand, things too wonderful for me to know.' Like Job, I am compelled to say, 'Therefore I despise myself and repent.' I am your servant."

"My son, I still have work for you to finish here on earth. However your remaining days in this body are few. Many people, those who you have touched, will soon come to you. You will bless them and they will help you further understand the impact of your life. Here on earth I have many capstone children and you are one. If you remove the capstone, the building will crumble. If you remove a capstone child, my plan for blessing and salvation will fail. However be confident of this, my plans will never fail.

Frank, be strong and courageous, be full of hope and anticipation for it is written:

"No eye has seen
No ear has heard,
No mind has conceived
What God has prepared for
Those who love him." (I Co. 2:9)

Praise God that he reveals his truths to man. Encouraged, I felt strengthened as never before. Truly, God's power was being made perfect in my weakness. Even though my body was not capable of moving, the power of the Holy Spirit was unstoppable.

Time and the world began to return to as it had been. Nurse Inez Perkins walked into my room. She looked at me without speaking. She went through her checklist of the things she was supposed to do for me in her usual uncaring gruff fashion. The Holy Spirit spoke to my mind, "Tell her Jesus loves her and that you love her." Immediately, I tried to obey the Spirit but when I opened my mouth to speak there was no strength in my vocal cords. I prayed, "Lord, give my voice the strength to witness for you." Once again, I opened my mouth to speak but no strength was there to audibly tell her that Jesus loves her. In my mind I pleaded with the Lord, "Give me the strength for Nurse Perkins sake and so that you will be glorified."

Nurse Perkins could see in my eyes that I was trying to communicate with her. She gave me her attention and for the third time I opened my mouth to speak and said, "Jesus loves you and I love you!" She was startled not only by what I said but by the strength in my voice.

She stood frozen for a moment then she replied, "Frank, what did you say?"

Taking a deep breath, I repeated my message with the same power, "Nurse Perkins, Jesus loves you and I love you!"

She stared at me and tears filled her eyes. She continued her care routine but with much kinder hands. As she finished, tears rolled down her cheeks and without saying a word, she walked out of my room.

I knew the Lord was dealing with Nurse Perkins and that this was a critical time for her. Satan does not let go without a fight and he was sure to build those walls as high as he could to keep her from the saving love of Jesus. Knowing this, I spent much of that night in prayer for Nurse Perkins. No walls can be built that can prevent one who the Lord loves from coming to Him.

The next morning the Lord made it very clear that I was to repeat His message to her. She came into my room but not in the usual way. There was something different, softer about her. I fixed my eyes on her to draw her attention. In obedience to the Holy Spirit, I repeated His message, "Nurse Perkins, Jesus loves you and I love you."

It was as if my saying that again was that drop of water that burst the dam. She began to sob and she sat down on the chair next to my bed. Through her tears she said, "Frank, forgive me. I have been cruel and mistreated you and many others."

With the strength of the Holy Spirit I said, "I forgive you and the Lord Jesus forgives you. Do you accept Jesus?"

She lifted her eyes to heaven and said, "Please Jesus, forgive me and help me!"

Nurse Perkins began to unburden herself by telling me about the circumstances of her miserable life. The beatings by her husband, how he abused her children, her son who had killed a man during a robbery, she related how all her pain had made her hate everyone and everything. That is, until I reminded her that Jesus loved her and told her that I also loved her. "I never thought I would ever hear someone tell me that they loved me." She cried.

Nurse Perkins told me how, as a child, she always went to church and had loved the Lord. But she came to believe through the hardness of her life that God had forgotten about her. There is something in the spiritual world called "Divine Appointments." This was one such divine appointment. As Nurse Perkins was telling me the story of her tragic life, Ben McGraw walked into my room. Ben is a man who is very sensitive to the leading of the Holy Spirit. He immediately knew that the Holy Spirit was working in Nurse Perkins' life. After greeting me, he introduced himself to her. The Holy Spirit gave me the strength to clearly say, "Ben, she needs Jesus. She needs your help."

Nurse Perkins was called to another resident's room and had to leave but before going she promised to go to the Wednesday night service at the New Albany Church of God. Over the next few days I prayed continually for Inez Perkins. Her husband refused to let her go to church saying that he didn't want a bunch of hypocrites messing with her mind. I noticed a welt near her eye that she did her best to cover with make-up. She was in a bad situation and desperately needed help. I remembered the lessons about the Walls of Salvation. Certainly Satan was raising the walls around Inez to keep her away from God.

However, nothing is impossible for God. Ben McGraw was concerned and worried about Inez when she failed to come to the church that Wednesday evening. He knew there was a problem so he brought help in the form of our dear old friend Captain Judy Tortelli of the Salvation Army. Judy was very active in the community and led a ministry that helped battered women. Seeing Ben and Judy, I recalled the horrible possible scenarios from the life that might have been. I praised God for His unsurpassed wisdom in carrying out his plan for all of us.

"Frank, it's so good to see you." Said Judy as she kissed my forehead. Ben and Judy sat down in my room as we waited for Inez to make her rounds. While we waited we all prayed, asking God that he would free Inez from the prison in which Satan had kept her bound.

When Inez walked in and saw Ben and Judy, a look of fear came over her face. Satan was desperate to hold on to her and was doing his best to keep her in fear. Judy took her hand and said, "Inez, please don't be afraid. We're here to help you. I'm with the Salvation Army and with the Lord's strength I've worked with women just like you for years. I too was an abused and battered wife. You're not alone."

Inez replied, "Please leave me alone, there is nothing you can do for me."

Judy replied, "By ourselves that is true. But the Lord Jesus came to set prisoners free and he wants to set you free. He says he will never leave you or forsake you. You believe that don't you? Won't you pray with us right now for the courage to leave your life of bondage?"

Tears fell from her eyes as she nodded yes. Ben and Judy held her hands and began to pray for her. Inez began to shake as Jesus delivered her from the spirit of fear. Ben led the prayer and you could feel the power of the Holy Spirit as he rebuked the enemy. "In the name of the Lord Jesus, we rebuke you foul spirit of fear and subjugation, as the Philistine came against David with sword, spear and javelin, your power against Inez is useless and broken. We come against you in the name of the Lord God Almighty and nothing can stand against us. I declare this child of God free from your wicked bondage. I bring the blood of Jesus between you and her and serve notice that this blood line cannot be broken or crossed and we pray this in the all powerful and holy name of Jesus. Amen and Amen!"

Inez agreed to go with Judy to the Salvation Army's Downtown Women's Shelter after her shift at the nursing home was completed. When she didn't come home that night, Inez's husband showed up at the nursing home the next day and tried to bully her into coming home. I heard that when she refused, he pushed her. Praise God, Inez pushed him back. The nursing home security officer called the police and they arrested her soon to be ex-husband. Inez never went back to that abusive home. Indeed Jesus had set this prisoner free. A year later she was teaching a Bible study for women at The New Albany Church of God.

After Inez accepted Jesus as her Lord and Savior, everything started to improve at the nursing home. Inez was on fire for the Lord. She witnessed to everyone who worked there as well as the residents who did not already know the Lord. All of a sudden the quality of care improved by leaps and bounds. Those staff members who had previously been sullen and unfriendly were now loving and conscientious. Several of them even started reading the Bible to the residents.

I cannot take credit for the changes in the Inez's life or for the improvements at the nursing home. All the credit and glory is God's. But the lesson here is to obey the Holy Spirit. My human nature would never have said to Nurse Perkins, "I love you." But when the Holy Spirit told me to tell her, "Jesus loves you and I love you," great things happened. Indeed great things will always happen when you obey the Holy Spirit.

Thanks to the Lord, my life is better and it's a new day!

CHAPTER 25

THREE MEN IN A FOXHOLE

It was April 1st 1976. I had just been transferred back to the county nursing home after spending ten days in Albany Medical Center's critical care unit. I overheard the doctors say that the next bout with pneumonia would be my last. No matter, the Holy Spirit made it known to me that my time on this earth was almost over and I would soon be going home to be with my Lord. It was vital that I spend all the time my strength would allow in prayer for those I will be leaving behind. My sensitivity to the Holy Spirit was heightened and I became very aware that something unusual and amazing was about to occur.

The Holy Spirit never disappoints and later that week I had a visitor from the past, an old friend who I never thought I would see again. Nurse Inez came to check on me to see if I was able to see a visitor, someone named Johnny Canavi. My mind raced back to my last images of Johnny in the life that might have been as he reared back with the baseball bat, while being urged on to do his destruction by the evil Mr. Rizzi.

Johnny came walking in with a forced smile on his face. If I was able to stand, seeing him again would have knocked me off my feet. My heart soared, as I sensed that God was about to work a miracle. Johnny put his hand on my shoulder and said, "Frank, it's good to see you. I'm ashamed that it's been over fifteen years. I hope you are doing better. I heard you had pneumonia and just got back from the Medical Center. I guess I'm here today more for myself than anything. I hope you don't mind that I've come to see you."

I prayed for strength to communicate with him and to be able to speak coherently. "Johnny, praise God. I've never stopped praying for you. Do you have something you want to tell me?"

Johnny said, "Yes I do." He began, as he sat down next to my bed. "Frank, something is happening in my life. For the last week, everywhere I go and it seems everyone I meet is inviting me to go to church or is witnessing to me about Jesus. I've been a very bad man, especially these past fifteen years. I refused to stay in touch with you because, as I told people, all you wanted to talk about was Jesus, Jesus, and Jesus. People I haven't seen in years, like Father Matarazzo, do you remember him? He stopped me on Eagle Street a few days ago. Father M told me that he was involved with something called the 'charismatic renewal' and he invited me to a service he was holding in the old Leland Movie House. A day later I received a letter from David Greene. I heard that years ago he got religion and turned himself in to the cops. He confessed to these crimes he had committed that the police had no way of tying him to. I remember thinking he must have gone off his rocker. In his letter, he told me that he's been praying for me. He asked me to forgive him for how he tried to bully me all those years ago, and told me that he had a strong leading of the Holy Spirit to write this letter. He also included a letter addressed to you and asked me to personally deliver it to you. I guess this was his way of getting me to come and see you. "

I could tell that the Lord was really working on Johnny, that he was drawing him to Jesus. There was a calm sincerity about him that was very new.

Johnny continued, "Then yesterday I stopped at a phone booth to make a call and I found this on the tray under the phone." He held up one of those animated Gospel Tracts. "I found this cartoon about these three soldiers sitting in a foxhole during the war. One guy is a strong Christian and the other two don't believe in God. In fact, in the beginning of the story the three are at this military base and the two guys, who don't believe in God, are making fun of the Christian for reading his Bible. Sort of like I used to make fun of you; I'm ashamed to say. The Christian tries to tell them about Jesus but they just laugh at him. Later in the story they are in the frontlines during the war and are sitting in this foxhole and realize that the enemy is approaching. They realize that they are in for a real hard fight. Mortar shells are exploding and coming closer to them.

The Christian asks his two buddies, 'If you die today, do you know where you will spend eternity, Heaven or Hell?'

One of the guys tells the Christian, 'Shut up, there is no Heaven or Hell. When we die, we just die!'

But the other guy, realizing that they may not have much longer, says, 'I want to believe but isn't it too late?'

The Christian tells him that two thieves where crucified with Jesus. One of the thieves said to the Lord, 'Jesus, remember me when you come into your kingdom.' Jesus replied, 'I tell you the truth, today you will be with me in paradise.' The Christian soldier tells his friend that it is never too late to be saved.

The soldier then asks his Christian friend, 'How can I be saved?'

With bombs exploding all around them the Christian soldier asks his friend to pray this prayer;
'Dear Heavenly Father, I pray in the name of Jesus Christ.
I confess that I am a sinner and I now repent of my sins.
Please forgive me, as I now accept you Jesus as my Lord and Savior.
Please come into my heart, wash me with your blood and save me.
Please fill me with your Holy Spirit.
I will follow you for the rest of my life, trusting and believing in you.
Thank you for saving me.
I pray this in the name of Jesus.'

On the final page of the Gospel tract, the enemy storms the foxhole killing the three soldiers. In the last scene, we find the Christian and the believing soldier smiling and in heaven with Jesus. We also see the lifeless body of the third soldier lying and bloody in the foxhole."

When Johnny finished reading the Gospel Tract, I asked him, "Johnny do you think that tract was in the phone both just by accident?"

He replied, "No Frank, I don't. I think God put it there for me to find." I smiled, knowing that indeed this was the hand of God.

Then Johnny said, "Frank, when I read this story about the three soldiers in the foxhole, it made me think about me, you and Tommy. I heard that Tommy accepted Jesus before he was killed. I don't want to be that third soldier who wouldn't believe and ends up going to hell."

I asked Johnny if he wanted to pray the prayer of salvation in the Gospel tract with sincerity and accept Jesus as his Lord and Savior. He said yes. I asked him to hold my hand and to pray the sinner's prayer of acceptance. With tears flooding his eyes and his voice cracking, he did pray to receive Jesus.

"Praise God and welcome to the family of God!" I said with all the strength I could muster.

Inez walked into the room. She perceived what had just happened and started praising Jesus. Johnny asked me if I wanted him to read

David Greene's letter to me. I said to just leave it on the stand. I'll have someone read it to me later. I wanted this moment to be about Johnny. Before he left, Inez said a prayer that the enemy would be kept at bay and not be allowed to attack Johnny. It was very important that Johnny get involved with a church. He promised to go to Father Matarazzo's service at the Old Leland Theatre. As he was leaving, he vowed to come to back often to visit me. Nurse Inez promised she would check up on Johnny to be sure that he continued on the right path of his new spiritual journey.

A few weeks later, Johnny came back to see me. I wasn't feeling good and was very weak. Nevertheless, the Holy Spirit was telling me that Johnny needed my help and that I should rally what little energy I could. The Spirit told me that he would help me and give me the strength and wisdom to minister to Johnny. He looked very troubled as he sat down next to my bed. After some required small talk, Johnny got to the point of his visit.

"Frank, I am so ashamed. Just a couple of weeks ago, I accepted Jesus as my Lord and Savior, and I was doing real good too. I've been reading my Bible and praying, going to church and I've never felt better about myself. I even called my kids and they've agreed to meet me. Then last night something happened...." He said, then stopped in mid-sentence and just stared at the floor.

"Johnny, the Lord knows we are all sinners. That's why he came." I reassured him.

"I understand that, but what I did was real bad. Last night I stopped by the Elbow Room, it's a bar on Delaware Avenue. Long story short, I had way too much to drink and picked up this woman. She invited me back to her place and we had sex. When I woke up this morning, I just felt terrible. I feel like I let Jesus down. I let you down. I guess I'm just no good." Johnny confessed.

I replied, "Johnny, we don't become perfect as soon as we pray to receive Jesus. The enemy will tempt us and if we give in to that temptation, he then beats us up by telling us how sorry we must be. There's something called sanctification. This means that you are set apart for God and that the Holy Spirit will help you to become holy but it is an ongoing process. As long as you are on this earth you will never be perfect. The fact that you have such remorse in your heart tells me that the Holy Spirit has convicted you of this sin."

Johnny sat there and listened intently to what I was telling him. I knew that the enemy would love nothing more than to destroy this new child of Christ. I went on to tell him, "The apostle John told us, 'If we claim to be without sin, we deceive ourselves and the truth is not in us. If we confess our sins, he is faithful and just and will forgive us our sins and purify us from all unrighteousness.' I know you are sorry for your sin. All that you have to do is ask God to forgive you and he will. Pray for the strength to move on and overcome these temptations."

"Frank, I know that the Lord has been with you all these years and that he has helped you through but when you've had your worst times, your darkest days, is there a special prayer you say or a favorite Bible verse you read. What can you tell me that I can use in times like that." Johnny asked me.

I told him, "Through all these years, through the darkest of times and suffering, I always had hope. There was another man who suffered greatly. His name was Job. Perhaps no one in the Bible, besides Christ himself, suffered more than Job and yet he stated this about the Lord, 'Though he slay me, yet will I hope in him.' I have never given up on my hope that through all this there is a much better day ahead. Just have faith and always hope."

As I finished speaking, I could sense Johnny's relief. Forgiveness is a miraculous and wonderful thing. Johnny thanked me and after a little more small talk, he stood to leave. Before he left I told him one more thing. "Johnny, once you confess your sins in sincerity, God not only forgives you but he forgets your sin. He said, 'I, even I, am he who blots out your transgressions, for my own sake, and remembers your sins no more.' Man often says, I forgive but won't forget, but God in his mercy says, I will forgive and I will also forget…. So don't beat yourself up, OK."

With that, he laughed a little and said good-bye and promised to see me soon.

CHAPTER 26

BIG HENRY

Over the years, David Greene had written many letters to me. It always encouraged my heart to hear about the wonderful things the Lord was doing through David. In prison, David led many Bible studies, leading many prisoners to the Lord. He often wrote how both he and I were prisoners in our bodies but free in our spirits. Every other month a group of Christian men received permission to hold a weekend retreat at the prison. Ben McGraw was part of this group called the Kairos Prison Ministry. David always helped out and was even given the opportunity to preach at these retreats. He would also counsel and pray with the prisoners attending the Kairos weekends. David would tell me that many of the men signed up for the retreat just for the extra food that was provided and for a break in the monotony of prison life but many would leave transformed, having accepted Jesus as their Lord and Savior. One such man that David wrote to me about was a fellow they called Big Henry. Inez always stopped by my room before going home. When she came by I asked her to read me the letter from David that Johnny Canavi brought when he visited earlier that day.

Inez began to read;

Dear Frank,

I pray that my letter finds you well. Ben McGraw told me of your recent bout with pneumonia and that you almost died. I want you to know that I've been praying for you day and night. I too was recently in the infirmary. As I mentioned in my past letters, Satan has many disciples in this place. They think it enhances their status to attack a child of God. No matter, I continue to pray for them and as you know many have been won for Christ in spite of the hardships.

Do you remember me telling you about my friend Big Henry? He's the one who came to the Lord during one of our Kairos meetings last year. I am happy to report that he has been granted parole and will be living in a halfway house in Albany. I asked him to drop by and visit you. He is very anxious to meet you, especially after hearing about your struggles and how you have managed to overcome through the help of the Holy Spirit. Big Henry is quite a character and although he is still a babe in Christ, he is on fire for the Lord and is becoming a powerful witness. I know that his visit will bless both you and him.

I need to close for now. Be strong in the Lord my dear friend. I look forward to our homecoming with the Lord. What a glorious day that will be!

Your Brother in Christ,

David

David is such an amazing example of the transforming power of Jesus Christ. I am even more astounded by the grace of our God, after the Lord gave me a view of how we all might have ended up. I recall that scene from my life as it might have been and shudder. That horror of a night in the rain. The desperation of trying dispose of David's lifeless body. Thank God for his wisdom in sparing us all that horrendous life.

Inez put David's letter back in the envelope and placed it in a box we kept under my bed along with other letters I had received. I was encouraged by his letter and looked forward to meeting Big Henry. I remembered David's previous letter of several months ago when he first told me about this young man.

David met Big Henry on the first day of a Kairos weekend. Like so many of the men, Henry signed up for the extra food that was made available for the participants. Each participant was assigned a table to sit at during the group sessions. Every table had four men and a table counselor. David Greene was assigned to be the counselor for one of the tables. During the first session, David met with each prisoner assigned to his table in a private one on one session in order to basically take their spiritual temperature. David describes his first one-on-one meeting with Big Henry this way:

> I was sitting at a small card table when the biggest man I've ever seen walked in. I had seen him before in the prison yard and always steered clear of him. He was very intimidating and had a bad reputation. He had to be at least 6'7" and weighed well over 300lbs and was about twenty-five years old. My hands are not exactly

small but when I shook his hand it was as if I was a child. He sat down directly across from me and we were eyeball to eyeball. We introduced ourselves and I was real concerned that nothing good would come out of the session. He was very shy and when I asked him a question, he responded with a one or two word answer or just simply shrugged his shoulders. I managed to learn from him that he was in prison for manslaughter. He got into a fight over drugs and apparently he killed a guy with one punch from one of those huge fists. I thought to myself, he's just here for the food. My greatest fear was realized when we hit one of those awkward silences and ended up looking at each other as I mentally struggled for something to say. Fortunately, he spoke up first saying, "Shouldn't we pray or something?"

I replied, "Yes, that's a great idea. Let's pray."

I closed my eyes and started to bow my head when he said, "Shouldn't we hold hands when we pray. I've seen people do that before."

I was kind of nervous about this as it was just me and him alone in this small room, but putting my fears aside I reached across the table and held his massive hands. I began to pray, "Dear Heavenly Father, I thank you…….."

Big Henry interrupted me and now I was concerned that maybe I was in trouble here with this giant of a man. He said, "Shouldn't I be repeating after you when we pray. I've seen people do that before."

I replied, "Sure we can do it that way. That's an excellent idea." I was a little unnerved, concerned that maybe this big guy was just messing with me. But I began to pray, asking him to repeat after me, "Dear Heavenly Father," Big Henry was careful to say exactly what I said. "Lord, I thank you that you have brought us here together." It was about now when the Holy Spirit started to take over and guide me. I continued praying, as Big Henry repeated every word I said. "Dear Lord, I confess that I am a sinner and I am sorry for my sins. I ask you, Lord Jesus, to come into my heart." Just as I finished that last thought and as Henry started to repeat the words, I could feel his hands tighten around mine. He started to shake and I thought to myself, "He's gonna kill me!" But he stood to his feet and shouted, "LORD JESUS COME INTO MY HEART!!!"

The whole time we had been sitting there, the Lord was convicting him. I had never before seen anyone surrender to the Lord so quickly, so completely, and be so immediately filled with the Holy Spirit. Truly God had been waiting for Big Henry and there would be no escaping the Lord's call.

That concluded David's telling of how Big Henry came to the Lord.

Soon after, David sent another letter and told of Big Henry's initial experience as a new Christian in a hostile environment. The word in the prison spread quickly that Big Henry "got religion." Before this, nobody messed with Big Henry, but now some of the braver guys decided to test him. Immediately after coming to the Lord, Big Henry devoured the Bible especially the New Testament and especially the words written in red. He wanted to know what Jesus said and whatever Jesus said, Big Henry was going to follow Him exactly. "But I tell you who hear me: Love your enemies, do good to those who hate you, bless those who curse you, pray for those who mistreat you. If someone strikes you on one cheek, turn to him the other also." For Big Henry, these were words to live by and if necessary, to die by.

It started in the mess hall when one of the guys came over to Big Henry's table and purposely knocked his glass of milk over into his food. Everyone watched carefully to see what he would do. Big Henry calmly asked the fellow why he did that. When the guy laughed at him, Big Henry told him that he would be praying for him and tried to tell him about Jesus. In the world of prison protocol, that was the wrong response. The next day in the prison yard several men with scores to settle with the old version of Big Henry, attacked and beat him senseless, breaking several ribs and his nose. Big Henry did not try to fight back and spent the next two weeks in the infirmary. As soon as he got back into the prison population, he went to his attackers and tried to witness to them about Jesus.

Over the next few months he was beaten several more times, and each time the beatings were so severe, he ended up back in the infirmary and every time as soon as he was back on his feet he returned to his attackers to witness to them about Jesus. Eventually, they stopped beating him and began listening to what Big Henry had to say about the transforming power of his new best friend, the Lord Jesus. He invited them to come to David's weekly Bible study and several of them did and those that came ultimately accepted Jesus as their Lord and Savior.

So much of Big Henry's conversion mirrored that of his mentor David Greene's. It was as if the Lord had cast Big Henry in the same mold he made for David. As amazing and similar as both of their Christian awakenings were, it did not surprise me. The Holy Spirit is consistently amazing and he took two men in desperate situations and circumstances and overwhelmed them with the love of Jesus Christ. They both responded in the only way they could. So full of God's love and mercy, they were compelled to share this experience with everyone regardless of the result. Even if it meant being beaten or killed, it did not matter. This love of Jesus could not be bottled up, it had to be shared. He who has been forgiven much has loved much.

A few days after receiving David's letter telling me about Big Henry's parole, Nurse Inez walked into my room ahead of this mountain of a man. I was delighted to finally meet this man after hearing so much about him and about the devotion we both shared to our Lord Jesus.

"Brother Frank," he said, touching my hand as he smiled warmly. He continued, "I've been looking forward to meeting you ever since I've heard about your faithfulness to our Lord." Inez moved a chair closer to my bed for him to sit down.

I smiled back and told him how good it was to see the man I felt I already knew from David's letters. I sensed sadness in his spirit and asked him if he was alright.

He replied, "Frank, I'm afraid I have bad news. Our brother David is dead. They killed him in the prison yard." He broke down and started to weep for our friend as he told me this news. Nurse Inez was still in the room and she came over and put her arm around his massive shoulder to offer comfort.

He went on to explain that a gang of white supremacists had targeted David for assassination because of his work with the black prison population. "David didn't see color. We were all God's children in David's eyes."

I was saddened by the news and circumstances of my friend's death but knew where David was. I reminded Big Henry, "David Greene is in paradise with the Lord. Remember what Paul wrote, 'To live is Christ and to die is gain' (Php 1:21). David's journey and his work on earth are completed. His struggles are over. You and I will see him again someday. I believe that with all my heart."

Big Henry wiped the tears from his eyes and nodded that he understood. At the same time, I shared the pain he was experiencing. We talked for about thirty minutes until Inez came back to check on us. Because of the intense emotion of the news of David's death and the effort required for me to speak, Inez saw that I was exhausted. Big Henry stood up to leave and asked if he could come by from time to time to see me. I told him that I would be here if the Lord wills. As we said our good-byes, I knew that I would never see my new friend again. What little strength I had left was diminishing and the Lord was about to call me home.

CHAPTER 27

GOING HOME

It was May 13th, 1976. I often listened to a small radio in my room. It helped pass the time. There was a lot of talk about our nation's up-coming Bi-Centennial. Everyone seemed very excited and looked forward to all the celebrations planned for the 4th of July. It was different for me. I woke up very early that morning fighting for every breath. I was so susceptible to viruses and colds. More often than not, these colds turned into pneumonia. My immune system wasn't strong enough to fight off the infection. This one had come on quickly. My lungs were filled with mucus and my nasal passages were totally blocked. I struggled to breathe, believing that each breath might be my last. I was ready to be with the Lord but my instinct to survive kept me fighting. This continued for about an hour until Nurse Inez finally started her shift and came to check on me. She immediately called for an ambulance and they rushed me to Albany Medical Center. I remembered the last time I was fighting pneumonia, when I overheard the doctor say I wouldn't survive the next bout. In my mind, I kept praising Jesus. It was the only way I could manage getting through this. There is great peace in just saying his name. I knew that he was with me. Even with the respirator, time was measured in seconds and minutes, every breath was a victory.

I made it through that day and into the next. My family, friends and all those I loved were called to the hospital. I knew they had come to say their final good-byes. One by one they came, telling me how much they loved me and encouraging me to be strong in the Lord. I was unable to acknowledge their presence but was aware of what they were saying and aware of their tears. I could hear their prayers and oh how this blessed me, providing me with a blanket of peace. They wondered aloud if I could hear what they were saying, but they kept praying for me nevertheless and I thanked God for them.

My Uncle Peter brought my mother and father. She was now confined to a wheelchair. Ever since the time I was moved to the nursing home, she would come to see me as often as her strength would allow. Peter pushed her close to my bed. She wanted to touch me. She lovingly caressed my head. Tears rolled down her cheeks as she urged me to "stay with us." Oh, how difficult her life has been. Surely God will reward her for her love and faithfulness. Even my father was crying. He did his best under very difficult circumstances. So what if he got frustrated now and then. His life was bitter. I certainly won't judge him.

Aunt Camille, her husband Charlie and Brother Anthony came in. They held hands and speaking softly, they prayed, asking God to comfort me and to ease my pain and discomfort. Camille was my mother's younger sister and looked very much like her. She reminded me of my mother's love and of her sacrifice those many years that she took such good care of me. Indeed Camille helped us out so much over the years. God Bless her.

Sister Judy and Ben McGraw encouraged me to be strong, reminding me that Jesus was also there watching. Ben sat by my bedside and read from the Book of Acts in the 7th Chapter. The scripture was about the first martyr, Stephen, as he was about to be stoned by the Jewish leaders. Ben read, "But Stephen, full of the Holy Spirit, looked up to heaven and saw the glory of God, and Jesus standing at the right hand of God." Ben encouraged me that everyplace else in the Bible when Jesus is pictured in heaven, he is sitting at the Father's right hand. But here our loving Savior is demonstrating his great love and concern for Stephen, who was about to be stoned. He was so concerned that he wasn't sitting down but he was standing. Ben said, "Frank, if you can hear me, know this, our Lord Jesus loves you just as much as he loves Stephen and he is standing and watching over you. He's in paradise waiting for you." I could hear Judy quietly weep as she gently held my hand and said, "Amen" to Ben's words.

Big Henry was there and read the 23rd Psalm and praised God for the privilege of knowing me. I'm sure David Greene would be so proud of him.

Finally, my old friend Johnny Canavi arrived. We had known each other all of our lives and had been friends for most of that time. For awhile, I had lost him but now I have him back as more than a friend, indeed he was now my brother in Christ. I heard that he had become part of Father Matarazzo's ministry team, praise God! He had been estranged from his four children for many years and now thanks to the Lord had reconciled with them. Our God is a God of restoration. Johnny sat down next to me and rested his head on my bed and whispered a prayer. As he stood up, he touched his fingers to his lips and then touched my forehead and said farewell. "Addio amico mio," farewell my good friend. When I get to heaven I am looking forward to telling Tommy about our brother Johnny.

It was night and the darkness of my hospital room was cut by the light coming from the hallway. My loved ones had all been sent home earlier in the evening. The song, "It Is Well with My Soul," echoed in my mind. Years ago, soon after I came to the Lord, I sang that song in church. The words of that beautiful hymn strengthened me through my hardest times. "Whatever my lot, Thou hast taught me to say, 'It is well, it is well, with my soul."

I began to pray, "Lord Jesus, if my work here is finished please take me home." I repeated this prayer over and over. Suddenly, I was enveloped by that brilliant light, even more brilliant than before. But unlike before, I had no fear, only this overwhelming sense of peace. The presence of the Lord was with me. Slowly His presence manifested into the form of a man. No ordinary man to be sure, he was magnificent. He was dressed in a robe reaching down to his feet and with a golden sash around his chest. His head and hair were white like wool, as white as snow, and his eyes were like blazing fire and when he started to speak, each word lifted my soul and strengthened my heart.

"Well done, good and faithful servant! It is time for you to leave this world and come and share your master's happiness!" Said the Lord.

I was awestruck and could only reply, "Thank you Lord, praise you Jesus!"

He held out his hand to me and said, "Frank, my son, arise and come with me. It is time to go home, to paradise, where I have prepared for you a mansion."

Immediately, I was consumed by incredible strength and vitality. All physical constraints were gone. I jumped to my feet and then becoming overwhelmed by the presence of my Lord I fell to my knees and held on to Jesus. He helped me to me feet and said, "Follow me."

We walked out of the hospital room into the hallway. But it was no longer the hospital hallway. Everything had changed. A brilliant light continued to surround us. The walls and floor of the hall were beautiful, beyond my ability to describe. So brilliant were the walls of the hallway that I was able to see my reflection as we walked. To see myself standing upright and walking was incredible, amazing, awesome and more than that, I was young and strong again. My hair which had been shaved off was now full and healthy as in my youth. But as wonderful as my transformation was, it paled in comparison to being with my Lord Jesus.

We stopped at a doorway and the Lord said, "My son, there is something I want to show you." He opened the door and I followed him. The door opened to a large stadium filled with thousands and thousands of people. As I walked into the stadium, all the people stood at once and began to praise Jesus. He motioned for them to be seated and he began to explain to me about this stadium and the thousands of people.

"My son, all of these people that you see in this stadium are here because of you. My children are connected by a common thread. Your faithfulness in your ministry led many to me. Those won by your witness and example, in turn blessed others and so on and so on. The trials and sufferings you endured in your lifetime were not for nothing. They yielded a mighty harvest. Again, I say to you, well done!" The Lord explained.

The Lord has been so gracious to me. He has shown me the fruit of my sufferings here on earth. Those closest to me have all been accounted for except my three sons. I dare not ask about their circumstances and their standing with the Lord for I trust in him and know that he is mindful of my sons. But he knows all things and he is so liberal with his grace that he favored me with these words. "My beloved, you are concerned about your three sons, Robert, Frank and Ricardo. I see an old photograph of three little boys as they sit on the floor. They are all looking up and are smiling. Behind these happy faces there has been and will continue to be much sadness. Their road in this life is a difficult one. Many obstacles have been placed in their way. But for your sake, they will overcome these obstacles. I also see a photograph with three men standing together. They have been refined by the fires of life and now come forth as gold. More than that you do not need to know."

The Lord turned and left the stadium and walked back into the hallway and said, "Follow me." We walked some distance as the brilliance of the hall grew even more intense. Even so, the light did not bother my eyes in fact the intensity only magnified the feeling of complete peace that surrounded me. We stopped at another door which opened as the Lord moved forward. We entered what appeared to be a reception room. A group of people mingled about enjoying a celebration. As Jesus entered, they immediately gave him their full attention and began clapping their hands and praising the Lord. Their applause was not like the polite applause that is required by good manners for some dignitary but it was genuine, heartfelt and inspired by great appreciation and gratitude.

The Lord asked me, "My son, do you know who these people are?"

"No, Lord, I don't. They do look familiar. Please tell me, who are they?" I replied, as I did not recognize them.

"These are your loved ones and friends who came home before you. They've been waiting for you." The Lord explained.

Those in the room formed a reception line and the Lord urged me to go and celebrate my homecoming with my loved ones. The first person in line was a beautiful young woman. I must say that I hadn't a clue as to who she was. I soon recalled that her encouragement in my life was very helpful. She hugged my neck and introduced herself as Eva Grantland and immediately I remembered that she was the wonderful 88 year old lady from the nursing home.

"Eva, you blessed me so much with your words of encouragement that day in the nursing home. You said to me, 'Frank, whatever happens to you, no matter how bad things get, just remember that someday you and I will get brand new healthy bodies. Someday, you and I will run and jump again. Don't forget that and never stop trusting God. Don't give up!"

She smiled and replied, "I remember that day well. I lived on hope and wanted to plant the same seed of hope that encouraged me."

"Well Eva," I said. "Just look at us now!" We were overcome by the Lord's faithfulness.

Standing next to Eva was a strong looking young man. "Brother Frank, I'm Michael. You knew me as Mikey, Peter and Estelle's boy." He said, introducing himself. "On earth I was bound by Cerebral Palsy. I was unable to communicate due to my disease however I did understand everything that was said around me. I accepted the Lord thanks to the family praying over me." He explained.

I replied, "That's wonderful and amazing. Our God will always make a way."

I immediately recognized the next man. It was my friend and partner Tommy Phelan. He looked like the young strapping athlete

I remembered from Schuyler High School. "Praise God for you!" Said Tommy, as he embraced me. "Welcome home Frank, thanks to your faithfulness to Jesus, I received the word of God and accepted it with joy!" He exclaimed.

"I am only a servant. I may have planted a seed but God made it grow." I replied. Then I told him the great news about our dear friend Johnny Canavi. "Nothing is impossible with God!" I exclaimed.

Tommy began to praise God with, "Amen and Amen! Isn't God amazing?"

Many more saints of God followed in the reception line. Most of them I had never met on earth. But they shared their testimony about how my letters had blessed them. All their stories were similar. "Faith comes from hearing the message and the message is heard through the word of God." The many letters I wrote always shared the word of God, the message God gives to all of us in the Bible. Seeds were sown by my letters. Others, people like Brother Anthony and Ben McGraw watered those seeds. But just as I said to Tommy Phelan, we were all just servants, God made their faith grow. I was proud that God could have used me as an instrument of his grace.

Needless to say, I now recognize that none of this would have been possible had I not had Multiple Sclerosis. The proud, arrogant man that I was would have lived his life for his own pleasure and gratification. I had to be humbled and stripped bare, so to speak, for God to mold me into someone fit to bring his message.

My reception was a joyous occasion. As I went down the reception line, Jesus stood behind me and lovingly observed this reunion, nodding his approval. When the last of those in line had been introduced, Jesus said, "Follow me, there is something else I want to show you."

We returned to the hallway and walked down to another room with a large entrance way. This entrance was beautiful, quite grand with its solid gold doors framed by blocks of marble. Once again the doors opened as Jesus moved forward. Inside was a magnificent residence, fit for a ruler.

Jesus asked, "Do you know where you are?"

I replied, "This is magnificent. Is this the residence of one of your apostles or perhaps one of the great people of the Bible?"

Jesus smiled and then said, "No my son, this is your eternal home. Didn't I tell my disciples that in my Father's house are many mansions: If it were not so, I would have told you. I go to prepare a place for you."

"Yes Lord, your words always encouraged me." I replied.

Then Jesus asked, "Do you remember what I said through my prophet Jeremiah? 'For I know the plans I have for you, plans to prosper you and not to harm you, plans to give you hope and a future."

"Yes Lord that was one of my favorite verses." I replied.

"Those words seldom apply to one's earthly future, rather to one's eternal future. I cannot lie. Your illness was part of my plan for you, my plan to prosper you, to give you hope and a future." Said the Lord.

Jesus said, "I am your King and you are my brother and friend. You are an heir of God the Father and my co-heir. Indeed you shared in my sufferings and now you will also share in my glory."

Overwhelmed by his grace and his glory, I began to praise him! Indeed the words of the Bible are true;

"No eye has seen,

No ear has heard,

No mind has conceived

What God has prepared for those who love him." Amen! (1Co 2:9)

AFTERWORD

It was May 16, 1976. I was living in the small southern town of Hartselle, Alabama when I received a phone call from my mother. She had remarried when I was just ten years old and continued to live in the Albany, N.Y. area. She told me that my father passed away the day before and said she saw the death notice in the obituaries of the newspaper. She thought I'd want to know, in case I wanted to attend the funeral in two days.

Perhaps that seems like a strange comment. "In case I wanted to attend the funeral." After all, it would take some doing just to get to Albany from Hartselle, Alabama, not to mention the expense. For most people that might appear strange, you would assume that a son would most certainly attend his own father's funeral. But it was a very understandable comment given the circumstances of our lives and my relationship with my father and his family.

I had not seen my father in a couple of years and then it was only for a brief visit to the nursing home where he was living. I, along with my wife and son, went to Delmar, New York to visit my mother and step father and her side of the family. Out of obligation, I went to the nursing home and brought my young son Zach. It was the only time my father ever saw any of his grandchildren. My mother's brother Tom, a strong Christian man, had gone to visit my father several times and urged me to come with him to the nursing home. Prior to that, even though we lived in Albany from 1971 to 1973, I saw my father once and then only because I was shamed into going to Albany Medical Center when my father almost died from pneumonia.

There was no contact between me and my father's side of the family, save a rare letter received from my father's mother, my paternal grandmother. After some soul searching, I decided that the right thing for me to do was to attend the funeral. I asked myself the question, "Would I always regret not going? Years down the road, if I didn't go, would I regret it?" Not wanting to carry that baggage into the future, I made plans to fly to Albany the next day. I would spend the night at my mother's house and then go to the funeral the following day.

I had not seen my father's family in years and even then I could easily count the times I ever saw them in my entire life. My father's progressive form of Multiple Sclerosis had made him an invalid for most of my lifetime. This made it impossible for him to actively seek a relationship with me. From my view, when I was a child, there seemed to be little cooperation between my mother and my father's side of the family regarding any visitation schedule. I honestly do not know, but even as a little boy, I remember walking alone by myself the couple of miles from my mother's house to my grandmother's house to see my father. I can remember not wanting to go. It was painful to see my father wither away with this disease. I had this dread fear that I would "catch" Multiple Sclerosis and become an invalid like him. Plus, when I was with my father and his family, I heard an awful lot about Jesus. Not the Jesus I knew as a Catholic altar boy, but a different Jesus, a personal Savior and this made me very uncomfortable. As I got older, my visits to my father became fewer and farther between. This was a source of great guilt and regret that continues even till today. I always entertained the fantasy that my father and I would have had a great relationship if only he hadn't gotten sick. I was not a Christian back then but my conscience was testifying against me.

Years later, I accepted Jesus as my Lord and Savior and began to study the Bible. To this day when I read Matthew 25: 41–45, I experience deep regret:

> "For I was hungry and you gave me nothing to eat,
> I was thirsty and you gave me nothing to drink,
> I was a stranger and you did not invite me in,
> I needed clothes and you did not clothe me
> I was sick and in prison and you did not look after me."

> "They also will answer, 'Lord, when did we see you hungry or thirsty or a stranger or needing clothes or sick or in prison, and did not help you?"

> "He will reply, 'I tell you the truth, whatever you did not do for one of the least of these, you did not do for me."

There's a scene in the movie "Field of Dreams," where Kevin Costner imagines meeting his own father, who he never had the chance to know due to his untimely death. His father was a baseball player and he returns to the realm of the living as a young man, full of life and vigor and in his baseball uniform to Costner's Field of Dreams. Costner's wish is realized when as a grown man he finally has the opportunity to play catch with his Dad. That scene is almost too real and emotional for me to watch, for as a boy growing up what I wouldn't have given to experience playing catch with my own Dad.

I was a jumble of mixed feelings as I arrived in Albany. It was always good to see my family, my mother's side of the family that is, the side I felt comfortable around. But I was nervous and filled with anxiety about walking into that funeral home and seeing the other side of my family. I kind of understood a little of what the prodigal must have experienced as he headed back home to see his father. My father and his family were devoted to Jesus and not being a Christian myself at that time, I failed to take that fact into account. I feared that I would be shunned or at best politely tolerated.

The next morning, the day of the funeral, I woke up to the sounds of a hard steady spring rain. I started thinking that it was a sign from God that I really shouldn't go to the funeral after all. As zero hour approached, any excuse to get me out of this potentially uncomfortable situation was a valid reason not to go. I borrowed my mother's car and headed off to the funeral home wishing I was going anyplace else other than to this funeral. I rationalized that I hardly knew the man. No one would blame me for not going. Nonetheless, I drove on as it continued a steady downpour.

The parking lot of the funeral home was packed, giving me yet another excuse to just leave. I mean, I did at least try to go. Unfortunately for me, I was able to find a place to park on the street close enough to the building to not be able to use that as an excuse for just going back to my mother's house. Opening up my umbrella, I walked to the entrance and found the funeral home was packed with mourners. I wondered if there was more than one funeral service being held.

As I entered the building, my heart raced in anticipation of being rejected. I wondered if my two half brothers would be at the funeral. They would probably be in the same situation as I and it might make the experience more tolerable. As I entered the chapel, I went to the back of the receiving line and soon was able see the open casket with my father's body. They put a new suit on him. Other than a few flashes of memory from my days as a toddler, I couldn't recall ever seeing my father dressed in anything other than a hospital gown. My grandmother was standing over his body and caressing his head with her hand as she wept. Her sister, my Aunt Carmella, stood next to her with her arm around my grandmother to offer comfort. I worked my way up to the casket and found myself alone with my father. Everyone else had found a seat as the service was about to start. In my imagination, I felt the eyes of everyone in the funeral chapel boring a hole in my back. Standing there, I said a couple perfunctory prayers, wondering what length of time was appropriate for a son to view his father's body. I began to walk to the back of the room hoping to find a seat far enough away from my relatives when my Uncle Patsy, my grandmother's youngest brother approached me.

"Johnny, is that you?" He questioned, as I prepared for the worst.

I knew who he was and replied, "Uncle Patsy? How are you? It's so good to see you."

To my surprise, he grabbed hold of me and hugged me so hard I almost lost my breath. He led me to the first row of the chapel where my grandmother and grandfather were seated. They were overjoyed to see me. Room was quickly made for me to sit beside my grandmother. She held my hand firmly and was not about to let me go. Standing, she took me back to the casket. "Doesn't he look wonderful, he's so peaceful?" She said, just barely keeping her emotions in check.

When we sat back down on the first row, I could hear several people behind us ask, "Is that the son?" They were surprised that I came but seeing how happy my presence made my grandmother, I knew that despite all my initial trepidation, I made the right decision in coming. Several of my relatives came up to me and all seemed genuinely delighted to see me.

I soon learned that neither of my brothers had made it to the funeral. In fact, I was saddened to find out that my oldest brother Bobby had died. They were sketchy about how it happened but apparently he either had fallen from or jumped off a bridge. Nobody knew for sure. No one seemed to know anything about my other brother Frank Jr.

The service in the chapel was brief but very moving. There wasn't enough space inside the chapel to hold all the people who came, so the overflow filled the hallways right out to the entrance. After the service, several people came up to me to tell me what a wonderful man my father was and how he was devoted to God. I was amazed that this man, who spent the last twenty years on his back as an invalid, had such a profound impact on so many people.

When it was time to go to Graceland Cemetery, I started to go to my car to drive in the funeral procession but my family insisted that I ride with them in the hearse. When we arrived at the cemetery, even more people had gathered despite the inclement weather. I remember that their Pastor said at the grave site, "To live is Christ and to die is gain" (Php 1:21). At the time, I had no idea what that meant. Now as a Christian, reflecting back on my father's life, I understand that his sole aim in living was to glorify Christ. Why else would he have fought so hard to live those many times he almost died from pneumonia? His aim was not personal honor, wealth, pleasure even the acquisition of knowledge, it was to glorify Christ. Certainly he didn't fight so hard to live just to continue a life of suffering in a paralyzed body. When it was time for him to go home and be with the Lord, indeed for him, "to die was gain." In heaven there would be no more sin, no more questioning about his condition and his suffering with Multiple Sclerosis, no more anxiety and no temptation. To die meant to trade all those terrible things for a mansion of light and life, for peace, joy, comfort and perfect rest.

When it was time to leave the cemetery, my grandmother insisted that I return with them to her home to eat and to spend some time with them. The food was great but the blessing of getting to know the other side of my family was wonderful. I wondered how I could have been so anxious about going and what I would have missed if I let the negative human side of my personality rule my actions.

In the telling of his story, I mentioned a Bible given to me by my father as a Christmas present. I was probably 8 or 9 years old at the time. My father and grandparents had very little money but they went to the expense of having my name engraved in gold on the black Bible cover. I can remember at the time being very disappointed that I didn't receive a toy or something I really wanted. I tried not to show my disappointment but I'm afraid I didn't do a very good job of concealing my feelings. It is more than 50 years since I received that Bible and today it is one of my prized possessions. When I go to be with the Lord, I intend on leaving that Bible, the one I didn't want so many years ago, to one of my sons.

I deeply regret not making the effort over the years to know these people, especially my father. Many years later the Lord would draw me to His son Jesus. I was blessed to be asked to minister in a local nursing home and also at a senior retirement community. Over the years I've had the opportunity to tell my father's story at many chapel services. After these services, many people have come up to me to tell me how his story inspired them. Now all these years after his death, his faithfulness in living to glorify the Lord is still blessing others. Frank was the perfect example of the famous quote from St. Francis of Assisi, "Preach the Gospel at all times and when necessary use words." Amen.